THE
YOUNG SKIN
DIET

THE
YOUNG SKIN
DIET

Science-Based Recipes & Treatments
to Reveal Your Best Skin Ever

MICHELLE LEE

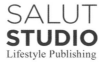

SALUT
STUDIO
Lifestyle Publishing

SALUT
STUDIO
Lifestyle Publishing

5200 Meadows Road, Suite 150
Lake Oswego, Oregon 97035
www.salutstudio.com
E-mail: contact@salutstudio.com

Distributed by Cardinal Publishers Group
2402 North Shadeland Avenue, Suite A
Indianapolis, Indiana 46219
800.296.0481 • Fax 317.352.8202
www.cardinalpub.com

10 9 8 7 6 5 4 3 2 1

Library of Congress Control Number: 2015915240
ISBN 978-0-9908817-2-8

Photographs of Michelle Lee by Marianne Wilson Photography. Food photography by Michelle Lee.

DISCLAIMER: The contents of this book are not intended as medical advice or to diagnose, treat, or cure any ailment, disease, or medical condition. While every effort has been made to ensure the accuracy of information presented herein and to accurately describe nutritional and other details of foods, ingredients, and other matter presented, The Young Skin Diet's contents are provided for informational purposes only. Your physician should be consulted prior to beginning The Young Skin Diet or any other diet plan. The author, publisher, distributors and/or retailers do not assume any responsibility for any adverse consequences that may result from the use of any information included herein.

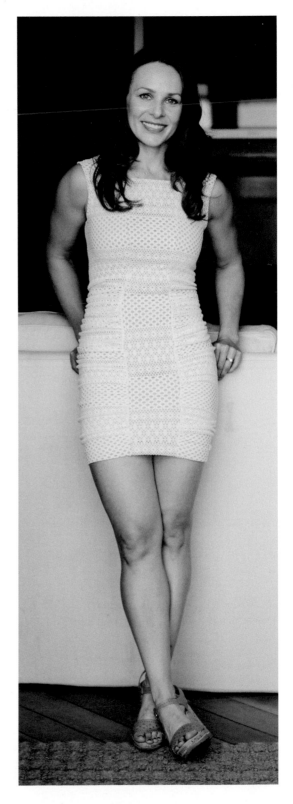

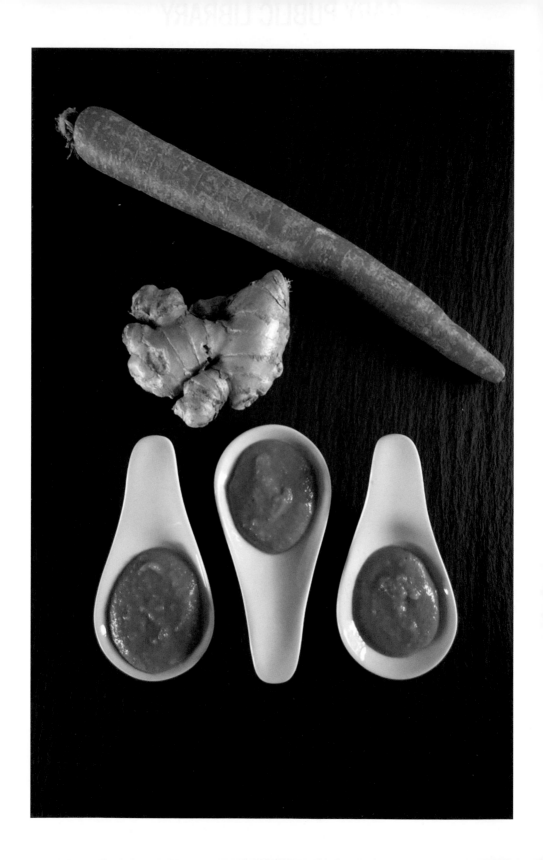

CONTENTS

THE YOUNG SKIN DIET

THE YOUNG SKIN DIET CALENDAR

BUILD YOUR OWN BREAKFAST GUIDE

BUILD YOUR OWN COMBO GUIDE

RECIPES

MORNING BEVERAGES

BREAKFAST DISHES

MID-MORNING SNACKS

LUNCHES

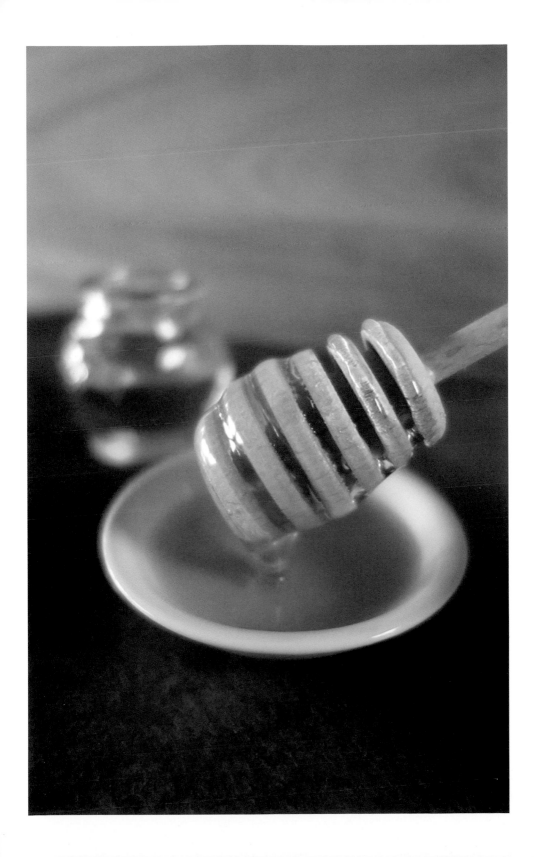

INTRODUCTION

The conventional wisdom had me convinced: Aging skin is simply a part of life. For all of us, fine lines, wrinkles, discoloration, sagging, enlarged pores and dryness at some point go from being distant future hypotheticals to very current, very real concerns.

I could see the effects of decades of sun exposure, stress and general fatigue on my face in the mirror. Where was that glow I used to have? More and more, it seemed to have given way to a compexion I hardly recognized as my own. I personally had gotten to the point where I felt like there was nothing I could do to improve my own aging skin without expensive cosmetics, products and treatments that offered only vague benefits with potentially nasty side effects.

What's the secret to young skin?

At an impasse about how to deal with the inevitability of aging skin, I turned back to the original problem. Was there really nothing else I could do to restore youthfulness to my skin? I thought about skin aging more deeply, and my mind was drawn to two important issues.

First, as an athlete and fitness enthusiast, I knew that regular exercise could render one's biological age much "younger" (by a decade or more) than one's chronological age. So if something as simple as exercise could keep our bodies young, I wondered: *What's the analogous natural and straightforward "treatment" for making skin young again?* (Exercise, by the way, helps a lot, but it's not the strongest weapon at our disposal.)

Second, as the wife of someone with food allergies and author of a book dedicated to cooking without allergens, I thought about all the people I know who have successfully addressed their digestive issues as well as acne, rashes, dermatitis and the like by eliminating common food allergens, such as gluten and dairy, from their diets. As I considered the topic further, I began to wonder whether consuming the right foods (and not consuming the wrong ones) was the simple, straightforward, no-nasty-side-effects answer to not only preventing allergic reactions but to halting – and even reversing – skin aging.

Hungry for answers, I turned to peer-reviewed scientific research to uncover the answers. I wanted to know, first, whether my general hypothesis was correct: *Can the right diet slow or reverse skin aging?* If so, I also wanted to know: *What, exactly, is that diet?* What I found was nothing short of fascinating.

To begin with, I discovered that I was on to something with my initial hunch. Our skin can be dramatically improved – made to appear younger – by eating the right foods (and avoiding the wrong ones), and the results have been tested and proven hundreds of different ways in dozens and dozens of academic journals.

Extensive scientific research proves the link between diet and rejuvenated skin. The Young Skin Diet derives from this research.

I also found that the science of skin – and the ideal diet for nourishing our largest organ – is highly intricate. It requires something more than just eating the foods often trumpeted by government guidelines and media headlines; while some of the readily available guidance on what constitutes "healthy" eating can be thought of as a useful starting point for dieting to improve skin, real young-skin results stem from more particularized nutrition.

In other words, **I discovered a large gap between the state of modern scientific knowledge regarding optimally nourishing our skin and the information we regularly encounter about healthy eating.**

Sadly, for all the good science out there discussing nutrition, skin health and the link between diet and young skin, there was not yet an easily accessible compendium of scientific findings on the nexus between our diets and our skin, and there was no satisfactory guide for translating any of that science into a real-world diet plan.

That's where The Young Skin Diet steps in. I've undertaken exhaustive research into the connection between, on the one hand, the health and youthfulness of our skin and, on the other, 1) foods in the diet, 2) combinations of foods consumed, 3) methods by which foods are prepared, and 4) when and how those foods are utilized.

I've distilled my findings into a real-world diet plan with recipes, treatments and tips that can be incorporated into anyone's life for tangible, no-nasty-side-effects results. And I've outlined things in a way that is not bogged down by overly-technical jargon and biochemistry – the findings are straightforward to understand and apply.

The Young Skin Diet is designed to make your skin young again.

In the sections that follow, you'll find:

- The Six Principles of The Young Skin Diet and why they are the essential foundation for ensuring your food works for you and your skin.
- Scientific research underpinning my recommendations on the optimal way to use food to make your skin youthful and healthy – smooth, bright, even-toned, resilient and supple.
- More than 75 easy-to-follow recipes and natural skin treatments that science shows build youthful skin, as well as meal plans, tips and food lists to make The Young Skin Diet simple to apply in the real world. It is in this way that The Young Skin Diet can be followed either as a comprehensive program as outlined in the meal plans and recipes or as a general roadmap with tools for dietary decision-making. These tools are provided in The Six Principles of The Young Skin Diet and in the provided discussion and recipes, which exemplify applications of these principles.

The science upon which The Young Skin Diet is based shows that dramatic results are achievable through the right type of strategic nutrition. Powerful research findings inform The Six Principles of The Young Skin Diet and the specific recommendations that are part of the diet. The following are examples of just a few of those findings.

- Healthy, middle-aged women who consumed foods that are part of The Young Skin Diet exhibited skin improvements including a 39% increase in skin microcirculation (i.e., bloodflow to capillaries feeding the skin's inner layers), 9% increase in skin hydration, 6% increase in skin thickness, and 16% increase in skin density. That is, the right foods can cause skin to exhibit physical characteristics of younger skin, and to thus actually become "younger" than its chronological age.

- The right food consumption patterns (which are part of The Young Skin Diet) can markedly and rapidly enhance skin pigmentation, for more attractive and youthful coloration and consistency.
- Application of topical treatments described in The Young Skin Diet improve elasticity and hydration in the skin by more than 150%.
- Foods that are recommended and incorporated into The Young Skin Diet have been proven to reverse UV damage, fight wrinkles, erase age spots and build connective tissue in the skin – that is they collectively cause skin to look and act "younger."
- When prepared and combined correctly, certain skin-ehancing nutrients are absorbed by the body at rates 500% to 2,000% greater than when otherwise eaten alone.
- Pro-skin nutrients can be chemically restructured to be more directly useful in the skin when eaten in the right combinations and cooked using the right techniques, as used in The Young Skin Diet.
- Proper food selection, combination and preparation strategies can ensure foods' nutritional benefits are synergistically, additively and cumulatively maximized for skin – which is part of The Young Skin Diet's scientific approach to using the diet to generate younger skin.

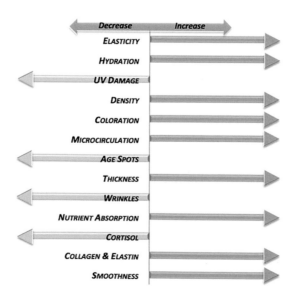

The Young Skin Diet: Effects on Skin

COSMETICS & SKIN HEALTH

Ingredients commonly found in cosmetics products, over-the-counter skin treatment goods and even everyday body cleansing products can have disastrous health and skin consequences. Parabens and phthalates, for instance, have been linked with increased cancer risks. Sodium laurel sulfate can dry and damage skin. Glycerin, too, can be damaging. This all still leaves unmentioned the multi-syllable, unpronounceable chemicals and pharmaceuticals often associated with skin treatments and "health and beauty" regimens, as well as the chemical cocktails that result in real-world usage of multiple cosmetics, skin care products and pharmaceuticals by a single person, as is generally the case. Many of these individual chemicals have catalogued deleterious side effects over even very short usage periods, and their impacts over the long term or in combination with other chemicals in common use may be entirely untested. The right foods, on the other hand, are natural – not manmade chemical amalgamations – that are well understood, are naturally "engineered" for coexistence with human use and have indeed been successfully used and tolerated by humans over both the short and long runs and in combination with other foods, for millennia. And, these foods can be readily optimized for healthy and youthful skin via simple, good choices about food selection, combination and preparation – without any nasty side effects.

To get things started as we embark on our journey to younger skin, I want to outline my philosophy regarding the search for answers about dieting for great skin since that search led to the bases for The Young Skin Diet and since it also distinguishes this diet from many others. I also will touch on my philosophy regarding my approach to ensuring The Young Skin Diet is engineered to work for you because, unlike many diets, The Young Skin Diet is specifically designed to allow successful adoption without major disruption to your real-world life. Following that, we'll dive into the science of skin, skin's relationship with nutrition, the particulars of eating for young skin and everything else you need to know to begin making your skin younger...today.

DIFFICULT SKIN PROBLEMS CAN BE IMPROVED WITH PROPER NUTRITION

I empathize with those reading this and thinking they have a skin condition that diet and natural treatments alone cannot address Maybe for some that's true but certainly not for all. Many who have suffered from eczema, acne, hives and other skin disorders have successfully improved them by eliminating gluten, dairy and other common food allergens from their diets. Moreover, studies show that increasing intake of certain foods can improve color, tone and composition of skin, while reducing inflammation, proneness to infection, puffiness, redness, wrinkling, sagging and dryness. The Young Skin Diet entails culling allergens from the diet and adding foods that are scientifically proven to not only make skin appear younger but also actually reverse the signs of aging. All The Young Skin Diet recipes are free from common food allergens and engineered to promote skin health.

I understand the importance of eating for healthy skin on a personal level because I have my own skin ailments that: a) I'm extremely self-conscious about; and b) I never thought could be improved by diet or natural means.

For starters, I've had rosacea my whole life. Growing up, gym class was a dreaded event where my skin transformed into a fuchsia mess that lasted hours after the fact. As an adult, rosacea has caused me embarrassing and sometimes painful acne and swelling. Happily, I've been able to manage and control my rosacea by following The Six Principles of The Young Skin Diet. And, because these principles are founded on scientific investigations encompassing results gleaned from laboratories and population studies, they're replicable. There's scientific research indicating they can work for you too.

My other skin problem? Melasma. While melasma has no cure, I've been able to eliminate significant portions of it and reduce other areas by following The Young Skin Diet's principles and by regularly using the recommended facial treatments.

Finally, I'll mention that I haven't always been a saint when it comes to skin maintenance. When tanning beds were cool, I frequented them more than I'd like to admit. And I've experienced my fair share of lobster-colored skin after visiting the beach on spring break or vacation. I also spent the better part of a decade living under the intense Southern California sun and more than a decade living and commuting in polluted cities like Chicago, Luxembourg City and Madrid. All those things have certainly taken their toll on my skin, and yet I've still been able to dramatically improve it through strategic nutrition.

It's never too late to make changes and see positive results – even when you think you've abused your skin to the point of no return. We all have things we don't like about our skin, and we all have the ability to improve them. The best part is that we can achieve improved, younger skin with something as simple as using scientifically tested nutrition strategies and natural topical treatments.

AN ANALYTICAL APPROACH TO FOOD & NUTRITION

I long ago abandoned trying to stifle my personality quirks. While it's true that some of them might serve me best if they were subdued a bit, one of those quirks has repeatedly proved itself worthwhile. That's the way I find answers to questions.

My approach probably is tedious, and in some instances I might be wasting my time. But it's just the way I'm wired.

Almost no matter the question, I have to find my answers in empirical data.

This means I'm one of those people who peruses the arcane journals and statistical studies that are the antithesis of exciting reading. No, academic journals are not the species of literature that keeps most of us up late at night flipping pages. And rightfully so.

Yet in their own way, peer-reviewed, scientifically validated studies are exciting. They reveal humanity's state of knowledge about a subject. They are often the leading edge of our grasp on the world around us. So I dive into those studies and distill my answers from what the research tells me.

Good science can provide the best answers to hard questions. I applied this philosophy to finding the best diet for young skin.

I turn to research because I want to see facts. I want to know, from bottom to top, how an answer to a question can be regarded as "truth." And I want to know the risks of that "truth" later being found false. I just don't have much patience for baseless assertions, untested theories or glossy packaging wrapped around specious claims. Give me statistical analysis, dry language and black-and-white graphs.

I'm an empiricist, plain and simple. No matter how compelling a notion may sound, no matter the seductiveness of a theory, I won't be convinced until I've seen good old empirical data that's the result of earnest scientific inquiry. That's how I find answers that satisfy my innate skepticism.

Part of this quantitative bent stems from my economics education and consulting background. Part of it is just my personality. But a big part of why I keep going back to the well of empirical data is the track record of success I've had finding good answers this way.

For purposes of healthily and sustainably improving my own skin, I decided to turn my economics training and empirical agnosticism to the science of skin health. After all, for more than 10 years I'd performed research professionally at the crossroads of economics and science, with emphasis on pharmaceuticals and medical technologies; I was dialed in to how to evaluate the merit and impact of research developments and how to form real-world conclusions and make decisions on the basis of good science. So, rather than use those skills to answer questions for clients like Fortune 500 corporations, I decided to direct them at understanding something more personally meaningful. Specifically, I was interested in answering a question: *What is the relationship between the foods we eat and the health and vitality of our skin?*

I wanted to find out if simple changes to my diet could lead to sustainably improved, younger-looking skin. I wanted to know the extent of good scientific guidance on which foods we should eat, how we should prepare and combine them, and when we should consume them for a more youthful complexion.

Through my research, which did include lots of nighttime page-flipping through academic and professional journals that refused to put me to sleep, I found answers. Really interesting ones, as it turns out.

I boiled down what I learned into simple, practicable guidance so that I could restore youthfulness to my skin.

Later, as I thought about sharing the results of my research, I wanted to ensure that not only would my essential question be answered satisfactorily for people interested in improving their skin. I also wanted to make sure that translating the science to real-world application would be straightforward to implement and easy to follow.

It is this line of thinking that led to the creation of The Young Skin Diet. It's designed to focus the soundest themes of modern science into a sustainable diet plan for improved skin. And it's meant to do so in a way that is real-world practical. No gimmicks. No specious claims or untested theories. Just good science, straightforward principles and practicable steps for your best skin ever.

What this means for us as we begin taking a journey toward healthier, younger-looking skin is three key things: 1) The Young Skin Diet is based in good science; 2) The Young Skin Diet's recommendations are derived directly from the research I uncovered; and 3) The Young Skin Diet provides a new perspective on nutrition for young skin. Here's a little bit of detail on each one.

The Young Skin Diet is a no bullshit zone.

If you're looking for "guru"-styled guidance on "breakthrough" (yet, unpublished and non-validated) findings about diet and nutrition, you can find that bunk in plenty of other places. Not here.

My research has revealed some compelling truths about nutrition and skin health, but none of it relates to Kirlian photography (seriously…?), alkaline/acid/pH dieting (come on), or other such nonsense. Unlike that sort of science fiction, the information you'll find here is validated, good, actual science (i.e., non-fiction) that can be very powerful in helping us achieve our goals.

My aim in this book, based on good research, is to help make clear what is and is not skin-friendly food, and how we can optimally prepare and eat those good-for-us foods in ways that fit our busy lives and restore youthfulness to our skin. As the science shows, the results of the right kind of diet can be dramatic and rapidly attained.

You will not be dazzled by research camouflage, citation overload, "conclusion puree" or study cherry-picking here.

Many diet books (if they bother to base their assertions on any research at all) contain hundreds or thousands of scientific-y citations that are relegated to indexes printed in size 4 type. And it's up to the reader to discern what research relates to which notions included in the book, leaving a vast disconnect between the purported research and proffered advice. Unfortunately, it's often the case that these citations appear to be included only to impress and mislead the reader, rather than to provide actual linkage between study results and diet recommendations.

Close inspection of the sources in such indexes often reveals that the cited research:

1. does not speak at all to the material conclusions of the book (i.e., the book camouflages empty promises with unrelated citations);
2. is cited despite inclusion of earlier or later study citations that more directly relate to the ideas (i.e., the book includes lots of research references simply to beef up the citation count: citation overload);
3. must be mashed up (or pureed) or, similarly, leapt from in great bounds, altering or abandoning the essential findings of the study, to link it with

proffered dietary recommendations; and/or

4. is marooned on an evidentiary island by itself, asserting a finding that is uncorroborated or even contradicted by the sea of good science contemporaneously undertaken on the same subject (i.e., it's cherry-picked).

Every food selection, preparation, combination, treatment and recipe I recommend in The Young Skin Diet is supported by an abundance of good science. I point to specific studies in each recipe that link the ingredients, preparations and combinations with young skin outcomes. And the study citations given in support of each are, indeed, relevant and useful reflections of modern scientific inquiry. So if a citation is included in this book, that's because, based on my review of hundreds and hundreds of published articles adhering to peer-reviewed scientific standards, I've determined that the cited study or article is both directly applicable in this book's context and likely to be helpful for this book's readers should further information on a topic be desired. "Helpfulness" is my own subjective notion here, but it is based on my assessment that the cited articles:

1. provide conclusions that are readily understandable, thus offering meaningful follow-on reading for those so inclined;

2. reflect the general state or direction of scholarship connected with the ideas explored, so the articles' findings are generally consistent with other good scholarship in the field;

3. review relevant literature in such way that is beneficial in elucidating useful background on the subject at hand, so the connections between earlier research and new findings are made clear;

4. proffer study results that can be linked to real-world-applicable suggestions and recommendations for eating to support skin health and youthfulness; and

5. do all the foregoing in such way as to obviate the need for multiple other citations relating to the same general conclusions.

Accordingly, in The Young Skin Diet, I'm not taking a single study or two and then warping the conclusions of science to defend some bizarre new feeding ritual. Nor am I hanging my hat on a single study, a couple of studies, or even many dozens of studies that present an incomplete picture of the landscape of relevant science.

Instead, I've looked to hundreds upon hundreds of studies. I've understood their intended scopes and their proffered conclusions. I've compared findings across categories of research and across methodologies. And I've used the full sweep of these studies to tease out certain threads that crop up again and again. Those threads, what I refer to as "themes," are the basis for The Young Skin Diet's recommendations

This means that a single, surprising finding in one journal does not have bearing on my recommendations. That is not to say, necessarily, that unusual findings can never be helpful. It simply means that, for me, there is not yet sufficient evidence that the unusual finding is "truth."

Concurring conclusions from multiple studies and multiple perspectives (i.e., those conclusions that all point in the same direction) do have implications for what I recommend we eat for great skin. It is these repeated, most consistent themes from good research that I regard as the validated, current "truths" we know about eating to support young skin.

Consistent themes from scientific research provide the "truths" about dieting for young skin.

As this implies, the aim of my review of these peer-reviewed empirical studies was to uncover the most important, well-tested and clearest prescriptions for eating to promote skin health and youthfulness. I sought to determine whether, from the current scientific literature, useful prescriptions could be made for how we ought to eat in order to better nourish our skin and rejuvenate it.

To perform my research, I employed all the skills developed in my training and career in economics, as well as my passion for health and fitness. Unencumbered by dogma that can come along with field-specific indoctrination, I stepped into the existing food science research with fresh eyes and skills attuned to digging through empirical research. I also did so with a predisposition to liking the research that employs good statistics and validated empirical methods, just as I did in my economics research.

This desire for quantification, measurement and validation powered me through articles published about food, nutrition, animal health, demographics, cancer treatment, human disease, sports physiology and the like. I found a robust field of study encompassing the intersection of food and health, with emphases ranging from sports to beauty to longevity to reproduction.

As a researcher, it is especially gratifying to find a field informed by so many outwardly diverse specialties since it means that many scientists are considering things from many different perspectives. That can lead to highly interesting and novel research, and it can set the stage for a deep understanding of those scientific "truths" I was after. This is because, when there are many perspectives involved and certain consistent messages still emerge from the body of research, there's a lessening risk that auspices bias, study design bias and other types of problematic (and difficult to root out) issues are confounding that field of study's conclusions.

So, the essential elements of a fertile research ecosystem were in place. If I could find repeated themes in the literature (i.e., those conclusions that arose in multiple studies conducted in related but not identical research specialties), I might be able to resolve those many studies' insights into a handful of clear points of guidance for great skin health.

It turns out I was able to find those themes and, then, as my research deepened and focused on core issues relating to nutrition and skin health, my study revealed increasingly practice-oriented, specific guidance. So, the research underlying The Young Skin Diet has two essential components.

The first is generalized background study that revealed "truths" or "themes" – principles which are discussed in detail in later sections of this book and which derive from the broad accumulation of knowledge I gained reviewing the literature. These themes cannot be attributed to any single study or research thread; rather, they are attributable to the collective substance of modern scientific inquiry's findings and emphases on the intersection of health, skin and nutrition. This first component of research can be thought of as the tide of knowledge in the field: generalized, encompassing and difficult to swim against. This is the basis for The Six Principles of The Young Skin Diet, and this provides the generalized guidance for using the diet to rejuvenate our skin.

The second is specific research guiding us on how those general and decisive themes may be practiced and optimized in the diet. This particularized research is called out specifically in each of the recipes introduced as part of The Young Skin Diet. These specific elements of research can be thought of as individual waves rolling into shore along the tide's broader push: They move in concert with the tide's advance and provide the explicit guidance we need to reach our goals for great, youthful skin as directly as possible. The findings of this more particularized research are exhibited in two ways in The Young Skin Diet. Most directly, they are found in the science summaries and citations accompanying each recipe. Each recipe presents a selection of science findings underpinning its link to young skin. More broadly, they are embedded into each ingredient recommendation, food combination, preparation technique, meal plan and recipe in this book. Even when not specifically cited in connection with a given recipe or recommended food, these findings manifest in every part of The Young Skin Diet. Just because a particular recipe, for instance, does not list scientific underpinning for each ingredient does not mean such science is absent; rather, it is found in this book. But to list such science again and again would be unduly repetitive and burdensome for the reader trying to keep track of it all. Collectively, the science presented in all the recipes outlines this particularized element of the research fully.

That's how I ensured all parts of The Young Skin Diet's cited research is:

1. directly related to the goals of improving our skin;
2. congruous with the best and most consistently observed themes in modern science literature on skin health;
3. easily and clearly linked with The Young Skin Diet's recommendations; and
4. clearly presented and non-repetitive in the recipes where enumerated.

The Young Skin Diet provides a different perspective on dieting and nutrition.

It is commonplace for consumers of dietary and nutrition research to glean information from news headlines reporting on a health study, from government-issued dietary guidelines, or from snake oil hawkers who populate the Internet with alluring misinformation (and flashy products). In principle, information-seeking is useful for people wanting to improve their nutrition and health, and I applaud news reporters and the government for their work to help us improve our lives through proper eating.

However, it often is the case that news sources disproportionately report either surprising findings (which later are shown controversial, if not altogether incorrect) or findings that suggest a "quick fix" or "superfood" approach to dietary enhancement. The news reports' headlines (e.g., "5 Superfoods You Should Be Eating Right Now!") frequently tout the new panacea food or seed or rainforest-derived wonder-berry while leaving out the context of that food's benefits. This is the nature of newsworthy material – those headlines do their job and encourage us to read on, after all – and so it is up to us news consumers to understand the headlines properly. Too often, however, in our busy lives, we just don't have the bandwidth to sift through it all.

The problem is amplified when snake oil salesmen pounce on the headlines' ideas and, in hopes of making a quick buck, repeat the ideas until they become "common knowledge truth" and the salesmen's opportunistic products sell, regardless of the quick fix's actual efficacy or the superfood's actual superiority.

Even in instances when the trumpeted fix or food really is very nutritious and beneficial, it is only as part of a generally balanced diet and healthy lifestyle that they'll do a body any good; these foods cannot be expected to materially benefit someone's well-being if wedged into an otherwise unhealthy context.

Thus, even the most well-intentioned information seeker will tend to be inundated with messages that suggest an imbalanced diet can be corrected simply by eating this "one great food" or by avoiding this "single problem food." Although it's true there are foods that benefit our health (and skin) more than others, a diet for good skin must comprehensively, holistically address nutrition.

The Young Skin Diet comprehensively addresses nutrition for skin health and youthfulness.

In other words, the science is unambiguous: There is no such thing as single cure-all "superfood," "trick" for good nutrition, or isolated change we can make for optimal skin health. **Real results come from consistently eating the right, strategic selections of natural, nutritious foods that are all in their own way "super" and, when prepared and combined with one another in the proper way, especially super.**

Similar in a way to news reports, there are government guidelines on healthy diet practices. Though admirable for their underlying goals, these also suffer from problems when it comes to outlining healthy eating. This is because most government guidelines base recommendations on outdated research, outmoded nutrition models or shaky studies that were influenced by lobbies financially interested in the shape of the food pyramid (or plate, or whatever we're using these days). There can be a gaping disconnect between what government resources suggest we eat for good health and what modern science recommends.

The two sources of nutrition information we regularly encounter in our daily lives accordingly have their drawbacks. Principally, they do not provide modern, comprehensive dietary guidance based on the full complement of scientific data at our disposal. And, for our immediate purposes here, they are not attuned specifically to dieting for optimal skin health and youthfulness.

My work in this book is to condense modern research into a user-friendly, easily accessible manual that we can all (enjoyably) follow to eat for healthier, younger-looking skin.

No bullshit. Good science. A new perspective.
That's The Young Skin Diet.

I've given you my philosophy regarding scientific truths and how those truths form the basis of The Young Skin Diet. Just as important, I want to address my philosophy in engineering The Young Skin Diet to esnure it works for you here in the real world.

I want to do this for one simple reason, and it's a sad one: Most diets fail.

The foremost cause of failure is that people simply stop following the diet plan before too long. Their stick-with-it-ness fades. And any health benefits achieved during the course of their time on the plan are quickly erased when old habits creep back into their lives.

If this pattern sounds familiar to you, you're hardly alone. According to a study done in the U.K., **40% of new dieters drop off their plan during the first week of dieting, and another 40% follow suit within a month**. Only one in five makes it past the four-week mark.

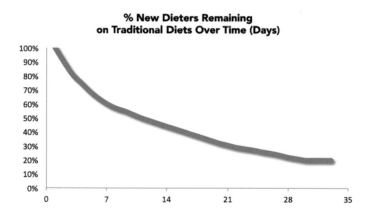

**% New Dieters Remaining
on Traditional Diets Over Time (Days)**

It may seem contradictory that 80% of dieters, who troubled themselves to undertake a diet in the first place, wouldn't see a plan through for more than a few weeks. *Why bother to begin at all?*

But there's good reason for diet attrition, and I've experienced it myself. When I tried the no-carb diet fad, for instance, I gave up in less than a week because I felt drained of energy, starved, and (worst of all for those around me) irritable.

Other diets impose unsustainable demands on adherents, requiring diligent measurements, rigid timing schemes or complex numbering systems.

Most diets simply fail to offer sustainable, useful, practical guidance.

In other words, it's not the dieter's fault for falling back into his or her pre-diet ways. It's the *diet's* fault for not recognizing that a sustainable diet plan has to be easy to follow. It has to become a seamless part of people's lives. It has to help people achieve their goals.

It simply is not enough for a diet plan to just proffer lofty-sounding principles or trumpet unrealistic programs. Those sorts of things may look enticing on paper, but they quickly become overwhelming in practice.

Nor can a sustainable, useful diet simply rely upon the take-my-word-for-it wink and nod of a nouveau celebrity whose blueprint for health rests on nothing other than feel-good aphorisms and dubious science.

Nor should we be satisfied by the circular promises, tortured logic and new age-y perspicacity of self-appointed diet "gurus." Their stuff's a bit too shamanistic for those of us here in the real world.

No, a real diet plan that can 1) actually be followed 2) for a sustainable period 3) by real people needs more. When I began thinking about The Young Skin Diet, I wanted to ensure it wouldn't fail people the way some diets do. I wanted to ensure it would be sustainable. I wanted it to be real-world effective. Overall, I wanted to be positive it would meet the essential criteria for a diet that allows people to succeed.

My philosophy is that a real-world-effective diet has to meet four criteria.

Based upon my review of survey results, conversations with real people who have struggled with diets and my own observations about diets I've followed (and attempted to follow), I determined that The Young Skin Diet would have to meet four criteria. I began referring to them as:

Science

Action

Results

Simplicity

The Young Skin Diet was designed with these four criteria in mind as means of ensuring this program won't let you down. Working our way down the list, let's first address "science."

1. An Effective Diet Has to Be Based in Good Science

Food and digestion are chemistry, biology and anatomy in action. Nutrition is not shamanistic. Guesswork is not a solid foundation for dietary guidance. The experience of a single person under some eating regimen is insufficient for programming the diets of other people. If we're going to commit to a diet, we need more!

If you're like me, you need scientific validation.

In this era, our society is blessed with empirical research that evaluates the macro- and micro-nutrient profiles of various foods, those foods' impacts on our bodies, the interactions that take place among foodstuffs consumed together, the biological implications of short- and long-term consumption of certain types of nutrients, and even the impacts of storage and processing on the things we eat and drink.

We often ignore this research at our peril, and many diet programs either disregard or distort the science and knowledge at our disposal. Such programs aren't designed with success and sustainability in mind.

A program arising from conclusions drawn in peer-reviewed scientific literature, however, does provide a framework for success since the input-outcome relationship is not conjectural or speculative or distorted but rather proved and replicable.

I'll discuss the findings of my survey of the scientific literature relating to skin health in more detail later on. But I will mention now that my review uncovered the presence of six strong themes in nutrition research that are overwhelmingly helpful in delineating what and how we should eat for youthful skin (and, as it turns out, healthy bodies).

So, yes, The Young Skin Diet is founded upon good science. **The Young Skin Diet adheres to the themes uncovered in my research and is engineered using established input-outcome relationships to help us succeed. Conjecture and speculation are left out of the equation.**

As good as scientific principles may be in educating us about what we ought to do, though, they're lousy at showing us how to actually go about doing it.

Sure, it may be interesting to learn that there are six key elements of diet and nutrition for great skin. But it's a heck of a lot more *useful* if, in addition to understanding those elements, we also have a plan for putting those principles into practice.

So any real diet plan not only needs sound scientific foundation. A sustainable and useful diet needs another key quality. It needs a practicable and actionable plan of attack: What to do *and* how to do it...gracefully. It needs "action." The Young Skin Diet provides actionable advice.

2. A Useful Diet is One that is Sustainable, Practicable & Actionable

What do I mean by "action"? I mean the principles – the scientific underpinnings – of the diet have to stand up to real-world conditions. The diet has to have a strong practical side that can be acted on.

How can we ensure a plan is practical and thus actionable and sustainable? How can we be sure well-intentioned people won't abandon the goal of having healthy, youthful skin after just a few days? There's a way, and it involves great taste, straightforward prep and real energy.

In sum, the action plan has to be simple to follow initially and easy to stick with. That means the foods meeting the diet's scientific guidance have to taste great. Meals have to be straightforward to prepare. And what we eat has to provide real energy to power a full day. The diet plan should not only be uncomplicated to maintain but hard to let go of!

The Young Skin Diet is designed to do just this.

Great flavor is, in my mind, the most important part of making an eating plan easy to stick with. Like anyone, I can't eat meals that I don't like for very long. I can fake it for a little while, but it's not really a sustainable plan for me to eat stuff that doesn't taste good, no matter the foods' purported health benefits.

I've never been a big fan of some fare that is evidently good for us, simply because it doesn't please my palate. Luckily, as I learned when writing *Living Luxe Gluten Free*, healthy food doesn't have to taste like "health food," so The Young Skin Diet's recipes are both healthy and great-tasting.

The Young Skin Diet's recipes align our flavor "wants" with our health needs. And, just as important, the scientific research indicating which foods, food combinations, preparation techniques, and consumption patterns are best for our skin (which I enumerate later on) can be applied outside of the provided recipes...and still yield satisfying meals. Following The Young Skin Diet does not require eating only the recipes given in this book; I'll show you how to make all foods you eat part of a flavorful implementation of The Young Skin Diet.

Straightforward preparation, like great taste, is another pillar of sustainability when it comes to actionable dietary advice. Nobody has an hour every evening for dinner prep. It's unrealistic to think we'll dramatically change our lives around to accommodate intricate diet implementation. If a diet plan asks us to do those things, it's destined for failure.

A diet plan should never *dictate* our lives. It should be the other way around: A diet plan has to *fit into* our lives.

The Young Skin Diet's recipes don't ask for much in terms of meal assembly, and preparation times are brief. For as little as they ask of us, however, they provide real results, real nutrition, real energy, and real flavor. And, the essential scientific truths these recipes are based on can be applied any number of other ways in easy-to-make everyday foods.

Real energy is critical to making a diet's action plan practicable. Like virtually everyone I know, I have a busy, hectic and sometimes overwhelming life to tend to.

Foods that don't keep up with my lifestyle are foods I don't have patience for. The meals in this plan are engineered to properly nourish the body so it can keep up with the demands of real life and also to enhance the vigor and youthfulness of skin. Indeed, the core food types that are most effective at rejuvenating skin also provide excellent overall nourishment, energy and satisfaction. So, in addition to sustainable, practical "action," the plan gets "results."

The Young Skin Diet sets forth sustainable, practicable, and actionable advice that is all results-oriented.

3. Good Diets Generate Results

If we're not getting what we want out of something, we'd be foolish to keep pounding away at it. Results need to be honest, achievable and maintainable.

The science of skin gives us useful parameters for setting out what is honest and achievable. This is because a person's epidermal skin undergoes renewal every 30 to 60 days, depending primarily on age. Think about that: Old skin gets entirely replaced by new cells every few weeks. **It's an honest and achievable goal for someone to eat for their best skin by properly nourishing and caring for skin cells as they proceed through the cycle of renewal.**

During the course of that cycle, there are ways to generate positive immediate results through good skin cleansing, exfoliating and moisturizing practices, even before old skin is replaced with new and properly nourished cells. Therefore, **included with food suggestions and meal recipes in The Young Skin Diet are "recipes" for natural facial treatments and skin care routines that help skin express its softest, clearest side, providing immediate results.**

This is a practicable and actionable way to have visibly improved skin within a week and for skin's condition to continue improving – getting healthier and younger looking – for the next several weeks after that. Indeed, the science confirms that many of the dietary and treatment choices shown to improve skin are cumulative in nature: their effects grow over time with repetition, rather than diminish.

The Young Skin Diet lays out the scientifically-grounded, actionable steps to make that happen.

Moreover, once the groundwork for healthy skin is laid, the benefits can be maintained simply by continuing to eat the right foods the right way and by continuing to treat skin as the large and important organ it is. The plan is sustainable. The Young Skin Diet is not a short-term, look-good-for-a-day-then-fade solution. It's a long-term solution to help you look your best – easily, naturally and happily – by providing real-world, science-based tools to achieve honest and enduring results.

I'll mention one more concept relating to results. A sustainable diet plan must generate the results for which it is designed without producing undesirable side effects. Some diets may provide the blueprints for weight loss but leave us drained and irritable. Other diets may be useful for fueling athletic pursuits but leave us imbalanced. The Young Skin Diet is engineered for great skin, but it also happens to be the case that eating for our best skin means we're properly nourishing our bodies generally – which can promote weight loss and improvements in body composition.

Everything in the program is designed to do a body good and achieve young-skin results. No exceptions. And everything is designed to do its job with elegant "simplicity" in a sustainable, practicable and actionable way.

4. Real Diets for Real People Are Simple to Understand and Implement

I'm human. I forget things. The last thing I want to do is crowd out important thoughts because I'm so worried about diet minutiae.

Rest assured that all the minutiae have been left out of The Young Skin Diet. **With this plan, we're taking on the big-ticket items that provide the biggest best-skin bang for our dieting-effort buck.**

The Young Skin Diet was designed so that it doesn't ask for much, but it does give a lot.

It's a straightforward program with clear connections between my research findings, food suggestions, the ingredients found in my recipes, the cooking and preparation techniques I recommend, and the prescribed natural facial treatments. The principles are simple to understand and adopt. The recipes are simple to make. And the plan is simple to stick with.

While on the subject of simplicity, I want to mention one thing about overly complicated diet plans. I've surveyed many diet programs, diet books and diet "gurus'" suggestions. I've found, more often than not, that guidance given by these programs, books and gurus is intentionally complex. Simple ideas that form the bases of these curricula are made labyrinthine in order to obscure their shaky underpinnings. There's none of that here.

In both design and execution, The Young Skin Diet is frank and transparent. I've worked to distill simple guidance from my review of many hundreds of scientific studies, to uncover themes from these studies that help simplify and optimize eating choices, and to keep the linkage between The Young Skin Diet and the underlying science clear and explicit.

In order to help keep things simple, I provide an easy-to-follow checklist of everyday habits and lists of "do" and "don't" eat foods to keep you on track without worry. Which means that following The Young Skin Diet – i.e., altering your diet to ensure everything you eat works for you to help make your skin younger – does not demand blind adherence to the calendar and recipes provided. Instead, The Six Principles of The Young Skin Diet can be applied through other means, including the use of my ingredient selections (found in my recipes and food lists) and the essential findings of science on the best combination and preparation techniques for those ingredients. My recipes and meal plans are intended to help make everything easy, but my overriding goal here is to provide you the tools to make young skin an easy everyday habit through information that helps guide good decisions. This is a "no-fail" diet plan because, so long as you can make small, smart changes to your daily habits, you can succeed in rejuvenating your skin.

our appearance by eating properly.

It is scientifically proven that we can eat for younger-looking skin.

Every food that is part of The Young Skin Diet has been vetted to ensure it will work for us to improve our health and skin appearance.

The combinations of foods, drinks and treatments comprising the program have been deliberately arranged to exploit synergies that scientific inquiry has uncovered. The whole of this program is worth more than the sum of its parts.

Cooking techniques likewise have been selected to keep more of the good and keep out more of the bad. Dry cooking of animal products creates advanced glycation end products (AGEs), which cause oxidative stress that degrades skin collagen. AGEs literally *age* our skin! By relying upon wet cooking and other basic insights of food chemistry (such as using the right spices and food combinations), we can largely avoid AGEs and unwanted collagen loss and can even provoke increased collagen formation.

And, the ingredients not included in The Young Skin Diet – things like processed and refined foods, excess sugars, unnecessary sodium, red meats and imbalanced fats – help enhance appearance simply by their absence. The diet also is free from common food allergens including wheat, gluten, dairy, casein, soy, corn and peanuts since they can exacerbate acne, inflammation, and other unwanted skin conditions as well as digestive issues (which can limit nutrient absorption and harm skin).

The Young Skin Diet is engineered to help us begin eating and treating our skin to support its function and, as a consequence, improve its smoothness, tone and color – that is, make our skin younger in appearance and healthier in fact.

The Young Skin Diet is engineered for healthy skin.

THE SURPRISING TRUTH ABOUT SKIN CARE PRODUCTS

Do you know how much money is spent in the U.S. on anti-aging skin care products every year? I'm not even talking about the full complement of skin care goods, cosmetics, treatments and procedures. Just those products aimed specifically at anti-aging skin care... Any guesses? Every year since 2010, consumers in the U.S. have spent a little more than $2 billion on this category of goods. For numbers geeks like me, $2 billion is right around the GDP, or the total annual economic output, of the entire Central American country of Belize. It's a hefty sum.

And you know what's even more surprising about lots of those anti-aging skin care products than their cost? Many either have no (or only dubious) scientific basis for any anti-aging effects and/or, worse, they include ingredients that are actually known skin irritants.

Yes, phthalates, parabens, sodium laurel sufate and glycerin are usually present in these products. For the vigilant, though, these chemicals have been on watch lists to be avoided if possible. But even seemingly innocuous ingredients – natural sounding ones – can be incredibly damaging and not benefit skin aging at all. Tea tree oil, for instance, is a popular ingredient in many potions claiming to reverse skin aging. However, the oil is known to cause allergic reactions including contact dermatitis (i.e., inflammation), redness and even blistering. I experienced this firsthand when I once bought a face wash containing tea tree oil, used it to wash my face before bed and woke up in the morning with a blistered face. My outbreak was so bad that it required a trip to the dermatologist and an expensive prescription treatment.

Other ingredients in commercial skin treatment products, including preservatives, fragrances and other chemical agents with ten-syllable, unrecognizable names, can likewise have troublesome effects on the skin, bulking up the chemical load our bodies have to deal with and thus causing misallocation of our body's resources.

All this is why I'm a proponent of external skin treatments using simple, natural ingredients with solid track records of beneficial impacts without side effects. The treatments I suggest in The Young Skin Diet are designed to both save your skin and your wallet from ineffective and problematic commercial skin products.

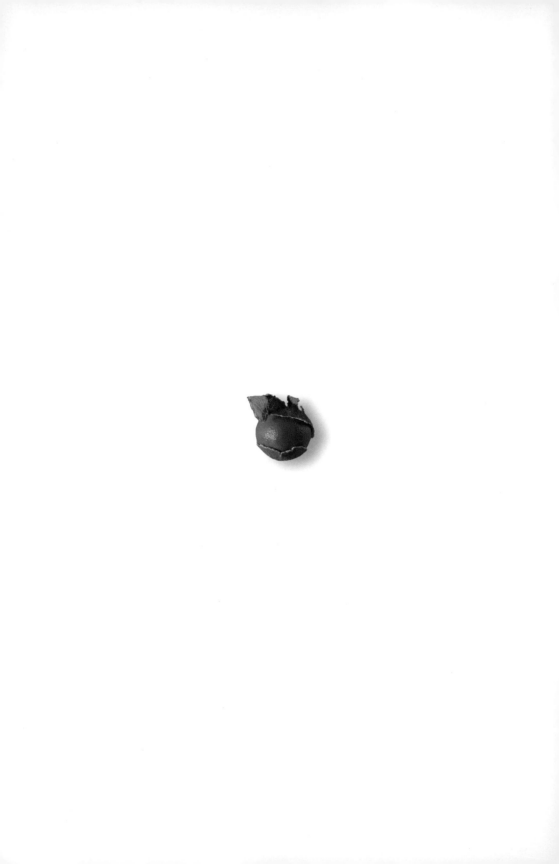

The first step in nourishing our bodies for a healthy, glowing appearance is to understand a bit about **our skin, the body's largest and fastest-growing organ.**

This organ is comprised of three layers, including the epidermis, dermis and subcutaneous fatty layer or hypodermis, which collectively provide a protective barrier between our bodies and the external environment.

The epidermis is the outermost layer and is made of keratinocytes and keratin. We tend to think of the epidermis when we colloquially refer to "skin" since it is what we most readily see and feel. Of chief importance in the epidermal layer (which itself is layered) is keratin, a very tough, fibrous protein that gives the skin much of its structure and durability. Over time, as we age, the quality of keratin cells in the outer portion of the epidermis declines. Damaged, old keratin cells result in rough and scaly skin, and the evidence of such cells increases with age as exfoliation action slows, environmental and UV damage accumulates, and nutritional needs are not sufficiently met.

The dermis lies beneath the epidermis. This is where collagen, a fibrous protein that imparts some of the skin's strength and helps tissues withstand stretching, resides. Elastin is the second protein complex found in the dermis, and, as the name implies, its chief function is to provide elasticity, allowing skin to maintain its shape following stretching, pinching and the like. Together, collagen and elastin are critical elements of the dermis that confer many of the characteristics we associate with healthy skin – pliability, suppleness, resilience and smoothness. Not surprisingly, the levels and rates of renewal of collagen and elastin fall as we age. And the protein complexes can be prone to calcification and reduced function along the way.

The dermis covers the subcutaneous fatty layer also called the hypodermis. It is generally composed of fat cells, connective tissues that serve a strengthening and anchoring function, and blood cell groups. Over time, the "plumpness" of subcutaneous fat underlying our skin tends to decline, and the capillary action (i.e., microcirculation) that feeds blood to the skin can be degraded.

Although the three skin layers work together as an integrated tissue to protect the body, each layer specializes in different tasks and receives nutrients differently, so each must be considered specifically in connection with dieting for youthful and healthy skin.

To that end, foods that are part of The Young Skin Diet feed the inner layers of the skin by supplying blood with nutritional elements that get delivered to skin by the capillaries. (And, foods that are part of The Young Skin Diet also have been shown to enhance capillary function and microcirculation to the skin.)

External treatments are engineered to tend to the outer layers of skin since they derive less of their nutrition from capillaries (which don't reach the outermost skin cells) and rely more on surrounding cells and the external environment for nutrition. External treatments also help advance the body's natural exfoliation of epidermal keratin cells, which ensures the skin's outermost layers appear as healthy as possible.

In sum, **The Young Skin Diet uses a two-pronged approach, feeding the skin internally and treating it externally, to help your skin be its healthiest inside and out.** This two-pronged approach results in immediate benefits and in long-term, sustainable, cumulative results.

This benefit escalation is partly due to our skin's state of constant regeneration known as cell turnover. Since skin cycles completely every 4 to 8 weeks, we can build better skin, cell by cell, through proper nutrition. In a matter of weeks, we can have a dramatically improved appearance and all the while we can optimize the health and appearance of our outermost epidermal cells with naturally beautifying and protective treatments. This is powerful since it means we can improve our skin both quickly and sustainably.

SKIN RENEWAL & APPEARANCE

If skin constantly renews, then why doesn't it naturally renew to reveal healthier, younger-looking skin? When new skin cells aren't properly nourished, metabolic processes don't work as well and our new skin cells simply aren't as healthy as they should be. Collectively, this leads to poor coloration, sagging and wrinkled skin that is more susceptible to futher damage from the environment. This ultimately leads to older looking skin following the renewal process rather than younger looking skin. With proper, strategic nutrition, however, we can turn the tables on skin aging and eat our way to younger skin, cell by healthy cell!

The Young Skin Diet is also additive and cumulative in nature – the internal and external treatments support and build upon one another over time for long-run increasing enhancements in overall skin health and appearance.

Illustration: Cumulative Benefits of The Young Skin Diet

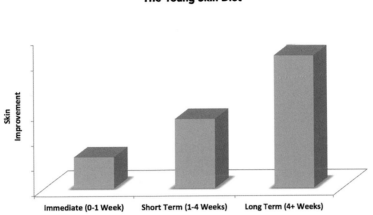

For instance, certain benefits of the external treatments included in The Young Skin Diet manifest immediately. Ingredients included in many of these treatments have been shown to result in skin hydration and elasticity levels around 150% of baseline untreated skin and to enhance hydration and elasticity more than 3 times better than moisturizers not using those natural ingredients. These benefits are realized within hours after application. Yet the hydration and elasticity benefits grow as the treatments are applied regularly over 3 weeks - instead of about 150%, the benefits grow to 175%.

Other external treatments exhibit similar immediate benefits, reducing inflammation and UV damage upon application. While others, with repeated usage over a matter of weeks, materially improve collagen levels and new collagen formation in the skin, resolve pigmentation inconsistencies, enhance skin color and improve microcirculation; that is, these effects are realized cumulatively.

Importantly, the biochemical pathways used by The Young Skin Diet's external treatments in providing these benefits are different from one another and from those used by the internal nutrition component of The Young Skin Diet. It is accordingly the case that they complement one another, each building upon the others' benefits, strengthening and rejuvenating skin additively, synergistically and cumulatively. Scientific inquiry demonstrates these positive relationships, so the empirical results of any discrete external or internal treatment given as part of The Young Skin Diet will understate the benefits achieved in combination.

It is nevertheless impressive to consider the power of certain internal components of The Young Skin Diet in isolation. According to one study, healthy, middle-aged women who consumed foods that are part of The Young Skin Diet over a 12-week period exhibited skin improvements including a 39% increase in skin microcirculation, 9% increase in skin hydration, 6% increase in skin thickness, and 16% increase in skin density. These findings are consistent with those of other studies I reviewed that demonstrate the power of strategic food selection and consumption for healthier skin.

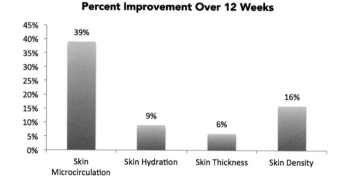

By way of further example, scientific findings indicate that even modest increases in consumption of the right types of foods perceptibly improve skin, making it appear healthier with more attractive coloration by 6 weeks.

Yet other simple daily dietary habits have been linked to improved skin elasticity, protection from harmful UV radiation, increased nutrient and oxygen delivery to skin and improved overall skin quality. Foods proven to provoke these sorts of enhancements are a cornerstone of the internal prong of The Young Skin Diet and they work to impart long-term sustainable benefits that complement the immediate and long-run skin benefits of the external treatments.

In other words, feeding our skin from the inside to resolve UV damage, restore hydration, improve elasticity and circulation, and enhance consistency and coloration does not interfere with or diminish the benefits of treating our skin from the outside to undo UV photoaging, improve hydration, enhance elasticity and circulation, and restore tone, consistency and color. Rather, they work together in The Young Skin Diet's strategic program. Additively, synergistically and cumulatively.

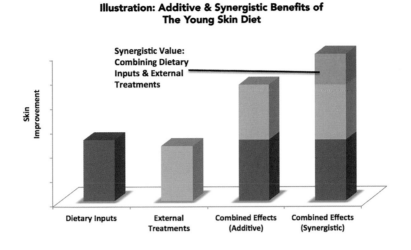

Illustration: Additive & Synergistic Benefits of The Young Skin Diet

Internal and external elements of The Young Skin Diet work additively, synergistically and cumulatively to promote a biological environment that builds and sustains healthy, young-looking skin.

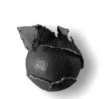

It's an unfortunate thing, but skin's flexibility, elasticity, strength, tone and texture can – and do – change over time and in response to external and internal stressors. We colloquially refer to these changes as skin aging.

There are three primary causes of skin aging: chronological aging, photoaging, and aging brought about by internal and external environmental forces other than UV light.

The Young Skin Diet is designed to combat signs of all three types of skin aging.

1. Chronological Aging

Chronological aging is intrinsic aging of the skin that occurs with the passage of time. No one can escape chronological aging's effects altogether: sallowness, dryness and loss of elasticity are programmed into our genetic hardwiring. But the rate of activity can be positively or negatively influenced by eating and drinking habits.

The Young Skin Diet makes use of foods and beverages that have been scientifically proven to slow or even reverse chronological skin aging's "symptoms" and to thus reduce the appearance of chronological aging by, for instance, prioritizing consumption of foods shown to improve new collagen formation and impede damage to collagen and elastin. In addition, balanced fats that help maintain subcutaneous "plumpness," as well as antioxidants and anti-inflammatories that keep cells working efficiently, ward off damage and help maintain hydration, are emphasized. External treatments that help old and damaged keratin cells be efficiently exfoliated also combat the signs of chronological aging by helping reverse the accumulation of scaly and rough skin cells.

2. Photoaging

Photoaging is exactly what it sounds like. When the skin is exposed to sunlight, UVA and UVB rays from the sun penetrate the skin all the way to the dermis and cause degradation of collagen and elastin, those ever-important protein complexes responsible for skin's shape and resiliency.

The rays also lead to decreases in production of things like retinoic acid, which is essential for keratin cell function and maintenance. These effects, among others, are what lead to photoaging. Photoaging symptoms include all those things we desperately hope to avoid like age spots, wrinkles around the forehead, mouth and eyes, spider veins on the face, and a leathery texture.

While the first line of defense against photoaging is preventative (i.e., wearing sunscreen and avoiding prolonged sun exposure during peak hours), we can still take other measures of protection such as eating a diet rich in antioxidants and using natural, topical treatments to prevent, delay, reduce and resolve the signs of photoaging.

With The Young Skin Diet, we combat the damage that's already been done and use foods to keep further damage from occurring. In this connection, along with foods that improve pigmentation consistency and build collagen and elastin, **foods with proven UV damage protecting and reversing effects are emphasized in the diet.**

3. External & Internal Environmental Aging

Other external and internal environmental factors such as air pollution, smoking, lack of exercise, poor dietary inputs like processed and refined and imbalanced foods, emotional distress, and repetitive facial expressions (like frowning or squinting at your smartphone) can also contribute to aging of the skin.

The Young Skin Diet emphasizes whole, natural and balanced foods proven to counteract cellular damage brought on by external pollutants. It also prioritizes ingredients and cooking techniques that resolve "cross-linking" and wrinkling that happens with repeated facial expressions, as well as foods that antagonize the hormonal responses to emotional stress which are linked with accelerated skin aging.

AGING SKIN IN POPULATION STUDIES

Studies of different population groups, particularly those clustered around the Mediterranean Sea and those in certain Eastern regions, unambiguously show that aging in both behavior and appearance can be dramatically slowed with adoption of the right dietary and lifestyle practices. In other words, even in sunny environments like the Mediterranean, where photoaging would be expected to intensely affect populations, smart dietary choices that emphasize the right foods can stall degradation of the body's systems. These findings inform certain elements of The Young Skin Diet.

With strategic food selection and preparation, along with targeted natural exterior treatments, the three primary causative forces of skin aging are blunted and, to the extent possible, reversed, revealing younger-looking and healthier skin.

So, for optimal and fast results that address the drivers of skin aging, The Young Skin Diet uses good foods on the inside to improve the quality of new skin, erase oxidative stress, enhance collagen and elasticity, and keep cells plump and nourished. And the program uses facial treatments on the outside to synergize with these internal efforts while also directly addressing the exfoliation and hydration action at the outermost layers of the epidermis where the blood supply does not reach.

Inside and out, the program is designed to provide the right balance and quantity of the most important inputs that our skin needs. It's arranged to ensure an ecosystem for healthy skin is maintained in the body's dynamic and complex systems, while fighting the onslaught of toxins and damaging agents found in our everyday environments.

More broadly, the foundational principles upon which the program is modeled can help us make better decisions at all times of the day, over the long term, so that the good we do for our diets can become an ongoing part of our lives.

The Young Skin Diet fights all types of sking aging, sustainably.

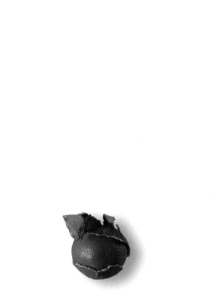

FOOD FOR YOUNG SKIN: CORE PRINCIPLES

In order to create the plan and recipes included in this book to combat and reverse skin aging, I examined peer-reviewed scientific journal articles focused on health, nutrition, biology, medicine, biochemistry, physiology, dermatology and related fields.

Many of the articles I reviewed discuss research into the biological impacts of certain foods on human health. Others describe the antioxidant, anti-inflammatory, nutritive, medicinal and other capacities of foods and those foods' effects on our bodies. Yet others detail population studies seeking to determine factors responsible for desirable (or undesirable) health outcomes.

From these types of studies I learned a great deal about the state of scientific knowledge on diet and nutrition. I also learned that, for every question answered about nutrition, several new questions arise.

For instance, while it is widely accepted that certain foods effect strong anti-inflammatory responses in the body, it is not always known why those anti-inflammation responses occur since the specific anti-inflammatory chemicals cannot be isolated or found to exert anti-inflammation effects in the lab. Similarly, while one study may establish that a certain phytochemical in a food is responsible for antioxidant activity in the body, another study will come to the conclusion that the phytochemical really only results in strong antioxidant activity in the presence of other phytochemicals.

It is accordingly the case that, as with any branch of growing and emerging science, there remain unknowns and areas for deeper inquiry. This is, after all, cutting edge science.

Notwithstanding the evolving nature of scientific knowledge, my research uncovered themes in evidence across the various journals and articles I reviewed that are well established, thoroughly tested and not prone to material revision as the science progresses.

As illustration of the concept, one overarching takeaway from my research is illustrated by the apparent contradiction found in studies relating to antioxidant and anti-inflammatory chemicals. Demographic and population studies evaluating health and aging unambiguously show that populations eating greater proportions of antioxidant-rich foods and foods with known anti-inflammatory action in the body have dramatically superior health outcomes – and are much more likely to appear younger than their biological ages would suggest – than populations consuming smaller proportions of these foods. There simply is no question about the dietary impact, and the studies indicate major roles for anti-oxidants and anti-inflammatories in driving the health benefits.

However, many studies evaluating specific antioxidants or anti-inflammatory chemicals, particularly through the use of engineered supplements, find contra-dictory or unclear results. It seems the quantum of benefits shown in the real world cannot be replicated in controlled laboratory environments. Or, some studies even indicate that "healthy" antioxidant and anti-inflammation supple-ments can hurt our health and appearance.

What's the resolution to this paradox? **It's simple: foods and their antiox-idant and anti-inflammatory chemicals work best – and benefit our health and skin most – when eaten as whole foods and when consumed in strategic combinations, using smart preparatory techniques.**

So, even with all the great science available to help guide our decision-mak-ing about nutrition, my top-down evaluation of the literature served as a constant reminder that everything must be viewed in context. Which is why my research process yielded just six – rather than hundreds – of guiding principles for opti-mizing skin's youthfulness through nutrition.

These principles are the thematic tides of good scientific inquiry. They re-flect the best and most consistent findings of science on how the diet can reduce and reverse skin aging. These notions rise above the particular conclusions of a single study or research thread; they are the repeated, confirmed "truths" that modern scientific inquiry reveals. They tell us, in general, how we can eat for younger skin, and they do so in a way that we can rely upon since these truths are so widely validated and corroborated across the many intersecting fields of study I investigated. These themes are the six principles for using the diet to give us healthier, younger-looking skin. These are The Six Principles of The Young Skin Diet.

THE SIX PRINCIPLES OF EATING FOR YOUNG SKIN

What follows are the six keys to a healthy diet supportive of youthful skin. These are the persistent themes disclosed in the studies I reviewed, and these keys to eating for healthy skin form the basis for the meal plans and recipes in my program. They also are foundational in connection with the external skin treatments that are part of The Young Skin Diet. More generally, these principles help us understand what we ought to demand of the foods we put in our bodies so that we consistently receive the dietary support we need for great, young-looking skin.

1. Anti-oxidation

Oxidation is a normal part of cellular metabolism. Metabolic processes in our cells release unbound oxygen molecules as byproducts of usual life-sustaining activity.

But these "free radicals," as we've come to know them, also are brought on (in more damaging proportion) by environmental forces including UV exposure and poor dietary choices. And this, really, is where the trouble starts. Unbound oxygen radicals are reactive and can cause problems for the body's cells and processes, and too many of them in the body can overwhelm us, essentially polluting the body's internal ecosystem.

In the aggregate, lots of reactive oxidation can result in premature aging, unchecked cellular reproduction (i.e., cancer), cellular damage and mutation, and a host of other problems that degrade health. **In the skin, excessive oxidation is responsible for premature wrinkling, age spots, sallowness, sagging, and other such signals that our body's ecosystem is being overly taxed.**

Too much sun accelerates oxidative damage. So, too, do excessive sugars, meats cooked at high temperatures, and refined foods. Metabolic processes that help the body manage UV exposure and poor dietary inputs put off high levels of oxidative radicals in response to the exposure and thus render the body susceptible to damage following, for instance, tanning or ingesting highly processed foods. The body simply does not respond favorably to these stimuli.

Foods like vegetables, fruits, olive oil, seeds, and some nuts, however, contain chemicals that, when ingested, scavenge unbound oxygen molecules in the body, binding with them and/or causing the body to eliminate them. That is, these foods exhibit antioxidant effects and thus help arrest the damage brought on by excessive free radicals. Some plant-based foods like oils and spices exhibit strong antioxidant effects even when applied topically to skin. (From a biological perspective, it has been theorized that plants hold high levels of antioxidants as means of protection against their own environmental hazards, including UV light. Plant based foods are accordingly the richest source of antioxidants available.)

Antioxidant-rich foods help the body function properly, protect cells from damage, and promote overall health on a cellular level. But different foods' antioxidants behave different in the body, with some exhibiting more powerful or direct effects in connection with skin health. The Young Skin Diet's recipes and treatments incorporate foods that promote antioxidant activity in the skin to ensure oxidative damage is minimized and long-run health (and skin youthfulness) is maximized.

One area of interest relating to antioxidants is: How much antioxidant firepower do we need in our bodies? Can we have too much?

Though there has been scientific inquiry into these topics, no guidance has been set for "appropriate" or "optimal" antioxidant intake levels. It would appear any such prescriptions are a long way off if they are ever promulgated. This is for a variety of technical reasons (including accurately measuring antioxidant impacts in the body), the diversity of antioxidants and their various effects on the body, and because there is not much evidence (if any) to suggest we as a population are at any risk of approaching troublesome levels of antioxidants in our diet.

My research has not uncovered any meaningful indication that we can have too many antioxidants in our diet, provided we eat varied foods yielding an array of antioxidant chemicals and those antioxidants come from whole foods and not supplements.

TOO MUCH OF A GOOD THING?

Note that eating any single food to excess may be deleterious to health, including antioxidant-rich foods. Carrots are a good example since they are very high in antioxidants and yet, if consumed at high levels, can cause cartenoderma or excessive presence of orange pigment in the skin. Moreover, some emerging research suggests that, among cancer patients, high doses of some antioxidant supplements can help cancer cells more than healthy cells and thus damage health. The main takeaway from these types of findings is that a variety of antioxidant-rich whole foods is most beneficial for our overall skin health.

Antioxidant supplements and imbalanced food consumption, on the other hand, are not so advantageous.

The best way to ensure a beneficial antioxidant profile in the diet is to strategically eat a variety of whole, antioxidant-rich foods, and to prepare and combine those foods smartly.

What do I mean by "strategically"? I mean basing food selection, consumption, combination and preparation on scientific results.

Regarding selection, some whole, plant-based foods, which The Young Skin Diet prioritizes, can be considered "best of breed" for their antioxidant profiles. Certain varieties of apples, for instance, including Fuji, Red Delicious and Gala, exhibit vastly superior levels of phenolics and flavonoids relative to other apple varieties – as much as 2 times the volume and concentration. These sorts of "best of" varieties are recommended as strategic selections since, in the case of apples, these higher antioxidant levels can be advantageous in protecting and building connective tissue in the skin. They are accordingly called for in recipes like my Collagen-Building Pomme Snack. Kalamata olives are similarly superior to other olive types for their levels and accessibility of antioxidants. Look for these and other "best of" selections in the collection of recipes in this book. To the extent possible, every ingredient selected for each recipe can arguably be called the "best of," based on scientific findings.

In the same vein as these "best of" choices, other foods' antioxidants exhibit strong additive and synergistic effects with one another – so long as the entire food (i.e., each of its parts) is consumed together. This is stragetic consumption. Unfortunately, the components of these single foods are often separated in the traditional Western diet. Citrus juices and citrus rinds, for instance, produce significant synergistic antioxidant interplay. The same can be said for banana fruits and peels. Eating all components of such foods is another strategic choice and is found in recipes like my Clarifying Lemon-Ginger Water and Collagen-Boosting Strawberry-Melon Refresh.

But it is not just single foods whose components yield additive or synergistic antioxidant benefits. The right strategic combinations of different foods do it, too. Many of my recipes use additive and synergistic multi-food antioxidant combinations for enhanced skin. My Erase-the-Photodamage Pretty Powerful Pasta, for example, combines broccoli, tomato, and olive oil which, when eaten together, intensify the foods' antioxidant and anti-inflammatory properties and enhance delivery of those goodies to the skin. (This recipe and my Rejuvenating Mykonos Mediterranean Salad also specify anchovies stored in extra virgin olive oil because of health benefits resulting from that storage medium.)

Similarly, the combination of unrefined coconut oil and sweet potatoes in my Procollagen Sweet Potato & Eggs recipe works to help the body metabolize vitamin A and provide an enhanced dose of antioxidants to the skin.

Still other foods, when eaten whole and together, allow for improved nutrient and antioxidant absorption. For example, a 2015 study conducted by Purdue University scientists revealed that consuming eggs (both the yolk and white) atop salads made with raw, whole vegetables improves the body's absorption of carotenoids and antioxidants, such as lycopene and beta-carotene, by more than 500%. That means more antioxidant absorption by the body, leading to improved free radical scavenging and age forestalling effects. My Photoaging Protection Quinoa & Vegetable Poached Eggs recipe, among others, takes advantage of these specific relationships to amplify delivery of antioxidants to the skin.

Other combinations of the right core foods also yield additive and synergistic benefits for skin. Any food combinations in my recipes have been engineered to exploit these relationships, and should you desire, could be used in recipes and dishes other than those given in this book. All the ingrdients in these recipes have been selected to enable synergistic benefits with one another. The food lists provided in this book also can be used to formulate other beneficial food combinations.

Yet other foods' antioxidant profiles are protected and enhanced by the right kind of preparation techniques. This is strategic preparation. Garlic, for instance, offers its strongest antioxidant punch when the clove is sliced and diced as part of its preparation. Kale and broccoli (and most greens) benefit from limited and low-heat (or no) cooking. Contrarily, spices often exhibit enhanced antioxidant action when cooked for a long period.

It is in this way, through introduction of a variety of antioxidant-rich whole foods into the diet and through selections, consumption patterns, combinations and preparations of foods that The Young Skin Diet ensures effective neutralization of excessive oxidative forces in the body.

Moreover, by migrating diet choices toward the good foods outlined in my meal plans, recipes and food lists and away from typical processed and refined

Western diet calories, the oxidative burden on the body is lessened. So, fewer radical-unleashing monsters in the diet, plus more radical-scavenging oxidative assassins in our meals, equals a much less polluted ecosystem, a much healthier body and much younger-looking skin.

↓ PROCESSED FOODS + ↑ ANTIOXIDANT-RICH FOODS = YOUNGER-LOOKING SKIN

The treatments I recommend for topical application to facial skin are likewise designed to deliver antioxidant protection. These treatments have the added benefit of being able to do their work directly on the skin, where they can combat UV and other environmental damage where it manifests its symptoms. My UV Damage Reducing Green Tea Mask is designed to combat UV-related photoaging, for example, while my Eliminate Free Radicals Olive Oil & Ginger bath relies upon phenols in olive oil, which are shown capable of permeating the skin (unlike many antioxidant molecules), to scavenge free radicals directly from the skin.

Though all my recipes, treatments and recommended foods exhibit beneficial antioxidant profiles, a handful of specific foods and food combinations with antioxidant benefits that are noteworthy include the following:

- **Anti-Aging Green Tea with Lemon:** Green tea's catechin antioxidants are potent scavengers of free radicals; however, they are not always absorbed by the body because they break down during the digestive process. **Lemon juice's vitamin C has been shown to protect catechins in green tea to enable 500% greater absorption of the antioxidants in the body.** Since consumption of green tea has been scientifically proven to enhance skin quality and reduce signs of aging (due to the antioxidant catechins), this is an especially powerful combination.

- **Make-Your-Skin-Glow Spinach & Eggs:** Tomato, egg, spinach and olive oil work synergistically in four ways. First, egg enhances the body's absorption of plant-based carotenoids, of which tomato is an excellent source. Second, carotenoid and phenolic antioxidants behave synergistically when consumed together (spinach is a rich source of phenolics), the effects of which are to amplify free radical scavenging. Third, the combination of tomato and olive oil in this recipe is beneficial since the antioxidant activity of lycopene from tomatoes is magnified by about 20% when consumed with olive oil. Fourth, **when cooked in olive oil,**

tomatoes' lycopene molecules restructure to be more easily transmitted to the skin. Among other things, these antioxidants are shown to enhance skin color, thus rejuvenating one's appearance.

- **Young Skin Curry Soup:** Red onions exhibit stronger free radical scavenging and lipid peroxidation-inhibiting results (i.e., they're better at preventing oxidative degradation of lipids that can result in cell/skin damage) than other onion types or even garlic. Ginger, cumin, coriander, allspice and cinnamon included in the recipe begin with excellent antioxidant profiles. But **the heating process that is part of the recipe preparation has been shown to significantly enhance the spices' antioxidant activity levels.** Collectively, the foods' antioxidants cleanse the body's ecosystem to support skin.

- **Calming Rooibos Tea with Lemon:** Aspalathin is an antioxidant only known to be found in rooibos tea. In combination with other antioxidants in rooibos, **aspalathin suppresses oxidation, inflammation and production of the body's "stress hormone" cortisol, which has been proven to harm skin, degrade collagen and cause excessive oil production.** Lemon helps protect tea's antioxidants.

- **Photoaging Protection Quinoa & Vegetable Poached Eggs:** The vitamins and antioxidants of romaine lettuce, tomato and quinoa behave synergistically in the body when consumed at once. Romaine and tomato are sources of the antioxidant ferulic acid, which helps stabilize the vitamin E from quinoa in the body. **Consumed together, ferulic acid and vitamin E's protective benefits against skin aging are 200% that of vitamin E alone.**

The Young Skin Diet prescribes antioxidant-rich foods to combat excessive oxidative damage and corresponding unwanted aging of skin.

In sum, following the anti-oxidation principle of The Young Skin Diet entails prioritizing plant foods by eating 6 to 8 servings of varied fruits and vegetables per day, consuming "whole" plants as much as possible, combining plant foods with one another and/or eggs, and adding spices to core foods. Recipes provided in this book give illustrations and additional scientific details of this principle.

2. Anti-inflammation

Inflammation results when the body's systems are in imbalance. It indicates that the body is fighting to restore proper function and, in the meantime, is redirecting resources away from their intended uses to do so. This sort of resource misallocation is unambiguously bad, taking nutrients and energy from skin-supporting processes.

In addition, inflammation of the chronic, low-level variety is believed responsible for a host of Western-society diseases like diabetes, atherosclerosis, cancers and even Alzheimer's. Unlike acute inflammation that protects injuries from further harm, chronic inflammation leaves the body in a perpetual state of distress and resource deficit. With inflammation, the body is not operating optimally, so health and skin both suffer.

FOOD & INFLAMMATION

Some have suggested that foods' inflammation effects on the body can be ranked by quantifying the foods' fat type and quantity, vitamin and mineral amounts, antioxidant profiles and glycemic index values, among others. Though intuitively compelling, this theory has not garnered commensurately inspiring empirical backing and has been criticized as not relevant in linking inflammation and the diet. With this critique in mind, it is nevertheless pertinent to note that certain foods with strong anti-inflammation rankings from these sorts of estimations do, in fact, have empirical research showing them to be anti-inflammatory foods. Coldwater fish are among these. The underlying mechanisms that cause some foods to be anti-inflammatory and others to be pro-inflammatory remain under scientific investigation, and, although there is some research linking things like foods' fats and antioxidants to anti-inflammation benefits, the relationships are complex. Which is why The Young Skin Diet prioritizes food and diet practices that have actual empirical testing demonstrating anti-inflammatory effects, not simply theorized impacts.

Refined foods, sugars, excess sodium, imbalanced fats, meats, and allergens all contribute to inflammation.

A glance at that list of pro-inflammatory foods tells us why so much of the Western population suffers from chronic inflammation and its attendant health problems. Those pro-inflammation foods are readily found in fast food restaurants, packaged goods, vending machines, and convenience store snack aisles. They're quick and easy to eat, cheap to buy, and – for biological reasons that have to do with humans' survival millennia ago – fill our bodies with short-run feel-good hormones. They're also incredibly destructive.

By placing the body in a state of inflammatory imbalance, we set the stage for the onset of long-term health problems that cause us to look older than we are (and which can be lethal).

But there are plenty of great-tasting and nutritious foods that counteract inflammation and its causes. I outline the four key anti-inflammation food categories below.

First, fish like salmon, anchovies, sardines and barramundi combat inflammation with DHA and EPA Omega-3 fatty acids because they restore the balance of fats in our systems.

Although the biochemistry is complex, Omega-6 fats often are pro-inflammatory, while Omega-3 fats either have a neutral impact on inflammation, are anti-inflammatory on their own, or are effectively anti-inflammatory because they help balance fat intake that is usually too heavy in Omega-6's.

Omega-3 fats are critical in the fight against inflammation.

The power of Omega-3 fatty acids as anti-inflammatories deserves particular attention since its role in our bodies is complicated and since the Omega-6/Omega-3 fat imbalance in the Western diet is so pronounced. As part of highlighting the role of Omega-3's, it is important to set forth some basics about these fats because clever marketers have managed to obscure the Omega-3 landscape a bit.

There are short-chain Omega-3's and long-chain Omega-3's. The "short" and "long" refer to the length of the chain of carbons comprising the fat's chemical structure. Short-chain Omega-3 fat comes from plants (and is known as alpha-linolenic acid, or ALA), while long-chain Omega-3 fats come from animal sources (and, depending upon the precise length of the "long" chain, are known either as eicosapentaenoic acid, or EPA, or as docosahexaenoic acid, or DHA).

ALA is important to have in the diet since it is useful as an energy source and since it helps balance our overall Omega-6/Omega-3 intake. However, for true anti-inflammation firepower, it's the EPA and DHA that are most critical. It is possible for the body to convert ALA to EPA or DHA, but, since the rate of conversion is estimated to be as low as 1 percent, the direct consumption of EPA and DHA is preferred. So, all those cleverly marketed seeds and plant-based ALA supplements must be viewed contextually. **And emphasis in a diet engineered for great, youthful skin should be placed on long-chain Omega-3's.**

With that said, it is imperative to understand how much of those Omega-3's we ought to be consuming. There is the glib answer first: a heck of a lot more. And there is the more science-y answer: enough so that, given a healthy total amount of fat in the diet, our Omega-3 fat consumption approaches the level of our Omega-6 fat consumption. **The bottom line is we want something like balance between Omega-3's and Omega-6's.**

According to some, we ought to be shooting for a ratio of 1:1, though other findings imply that Omega-6/Omega-3 ratios of 3 to 5 are the threshold at which major health benefits become realized. Whether a ratio of 1 or 3 or 5 is just right is not all that important. What is important is that we get our Omega-6/Omega-3 ratio down from where it tends to be for most. Since most Western diets are estimated to have an Omega-6/Omega-3 ratio of around 15 to 20, getting anywhere close to even 5 requires some serious rejiggering of what we eat. (What would happen if our Omega-3 fat intake were chronically much higher than our Omega-6 intake? That also would be sub-optimal. Balance is the key here.)

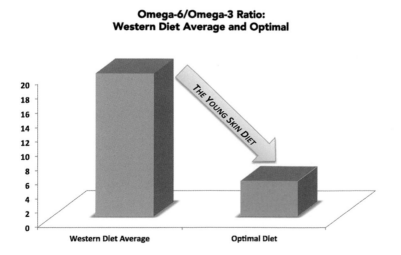

**Omega-6/Omega-3 Ratio:
Western Diet Average and Optimal**

The dietary rejiggering work is worth it. Getting our ratio down is associated with significant health benefits, like warding off colorectal cancer, breast cancer, cardiovascular disease, and asthma. Oh, and building great skin. Indeed, Omega-3's are responsible for keeping skin cells "plump" and helping maintain a healthy subcutaneous lipid layer that enables skin to have a desirable, youthful volume and shape.

The Young Skin Diet takes away the processed foods that contribute grossly imbalanced fats (i.e., way too much Omega-6 and virtually no Omega-3 fat) to our diet and introduces great-tasting foods emphasizing Omega-3 fats in a balanced presentation with Omega-6 fats.

Following The Young Skin Diet means eliminating (or at least significantly reducing) processed foods - no fast foods, packaged chips and the like. If you can't kill it, you shouldn't eat it. (Though not everything that can be killed should be eaten!)

The Young Skin Diet's Omega-3's come from plants as ALA and from animal sources as EPA and DHA. Among the animal sources most relied upon in The Young Skin Diet are eggs fortified with EPA and DHA, salmon, anchovies and barramundi (a wonderful fish from Australia also known as Asian Sea Bass).

Omega-3's per 100g wild salmon, cooked	DHA (g)	EPA (g)	DHA+EPA (g)
Chinook (King) Salmon	0.727	1.01	1.737
Chum Salmon	0.505	0.299	0.804
Coho Salmon	0.658	0.401	1.059
Pink Salmon	0.751	0.537	1.288
Sockeye Salmon	0.700	0.530	1.230
Others			
Sardine, canned in oil	0.509	0.473	0.982
Anchovy, canned in oil	1.292	0.763	2.055
Sea Bass, cooked	0.556	0.206	0.762

Source: USDA Nutrition & Your Health: Dietary Guidelines for Americans, Appendix G-2: Original Food Guide Pyramid Patterns & Description of USDA Analyses, Addendum A: EPA & DHA Content of Fish Species.

As with antioxidants, The Young Skin Diet is smart about Omega-3's. For example, wild salmon has an excellent Omega-3 fats profile and no meaningful health downsides, while farmed salmon is not so salubrious. So we use wild-caught salmon, as in my Anti-Wrinkle Spiced Salmon & Asparagus. Canned anchovies exhibit better retention and availability of their Omega-3's if stored in olive oil, so we use those rather than anchovies stored in other oil types (like soy), as in my Rejuvenating Mykonos Mediterranean Greek Salad. (These Omega-3 rich foods are more of the "best of" foods mentioned in connection with the Anti-oxidation principle of The Young Skin Diet.)

Recipes like my Anti-Wrinkle Spiced Salmon & Asparagus, Omega-3 Garlic Barramundi with Mushrooms & Wild Rice, Stress-Fighting Salmon Cakes and Erase-the-Photodamage Pretty Powerful Pasta are excellent sources of EPA and DHA Omega-3 fats. (Plus, the lemon and rosemary combination in my barramundi recipe has a synergistic effect in protecting skin from photoaging: It improves resistance to photodamage by more than half.)

Moreover, strategic combinations and appropriate preparation techniques matter in connection with Omega-3's. As with antioxidants, smart practices include the strategic use of spices (particularly "green" spices like rosemary, thyme, oregano and others), which help stabilize fats during cooking, as well as the utilization of protective cooking techniques, particulars of which will be discussed in detail later on.

In sum, Omega-3's are key in the fight against skin-damaging inflammation.

Second, vegetables and fruits provide potassium to offset excessive sodium, since potassium-sodium balance is critical for anti-inflammation. They also provide dietary water for proper hydration.

Excessive sodium is powerfully pro-inflammatory and is specifically linked with inflammation of tissues that harm the heart and can cause pain, while sodium-induced dehydration also promotes inflammatory effects in the body. All of this leads to premature skin aging.

By correcting a sodium imbalance and hydration shortage, skin can attain a more youthful appearance.

To combat inflammation, The Young Skin Diet's foods exhibit beneficial ratios of potassium to sodium, and the provided recipes collectively have higher levels of potassium than sodium – a stark reversal from the typically over-salinated Western diet, in which sodium intake grossly exceeds potassium intake levels, primarily because of processed food consumption. In fact, while most nutrition research suggests an optimal potassium-sodium ratio of a little more than 3 for superior health, most Americans' diets register ratios more like 0.7 - their ratios are completely upside down.

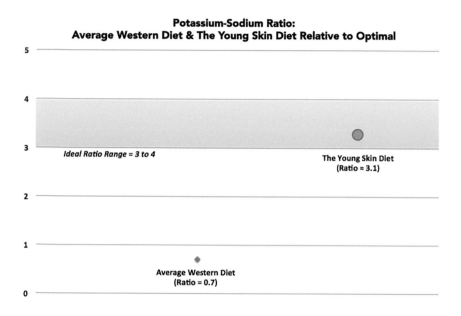

Potassium-Sodium Ratio:
Average Western Diet & The Young Skin Diet Relative to Optimal

Ideal Ratio Range = 3 to 4

The Young Skin Diet
(Ratio ≈ 3.1)

Average Western Diet
(Ratio = 0.7)

This is a troublesome long-term issue since the body's cell membranes rely upon equilibrium in sodium and potassium for sodium-potassium pumps to work efficiently in balancing the body's electrochemical profile. This is critical for efficient cellular function and youth-promoting health processes everywhere in the body, including the skin, where overall health is most readily observed.

All of which is why I have engineered the recipes included as part of The Young Skin Diet to provide the optimal ratio of potassium to sodium. Collectively, my recipes exhibit a potassium-sodium ratio of just over 3.1. In addition to this optimized ratio, the ingredients contain high levels of moisture to directly combat dehydration that can precipitate inflammation. The recommended foods given in the lists later in this book also collectively exhibit advantageous potassium-sodium ratios and, in varied consumption, can be relied upon to ensure a beneficial potassium-sodium ratio is achieved in the diet, even if my provided recipes are not specifically used.

An especially potassium-rich and hydrating recipe, among many others presented later in the recipes section of this book, is my Age-Defying Tropical Fruit Dessert, which features moisture-rich cantaloupe and honeydew, and a potassium-sodium ratio of 14. Recipes like this can help quickly remedy upside down potassium-sodium ratios and set your body's stage for great skin.

Not surprisingly, whole foods - as opposed to processed "goods" - are the best source for balanced potassium-sodium and hydration intake. Plus, these foods fill us up and help us avoid cravings for processed foods that leave us imbalanced.

Third, whole foods, prepared properly, fill us up with fiber and nutrients that reduce cravings for refined sugars, processed goods and other harmful, pro-inflammatory foods.

My Blemish Control Fruit Tea Cup is a "whole food" favorite for its great flavor and anti-inflammatory credentials, its beneficial fiber quantities and its naturally satisfying sweetness.

Whole foods are satisfying in ways refined foods cannot be.

But it is not just fruits and vegetables that provide whole food benefits. Certain foods that, in practice if not scientific categorization, we treat as grains can be particularly useful in imparting nutrition and satisfaction that quashes cravings for unhealthy fare. Quinoa, oats and wild rice are especially useful in this regard because of their ease of preparation and culinary versatility, as well as their fiber, protein and micronutrient profiles. Indeed, oats provide beta-glucans which are noted anti-inflammatories, and quinoa saponins have been associated with direct anti-inflammatory effects.

Various of my recipes outlined in The Young Skin Diet utilize quinoa, wild rice and gluten-free rolled oats, including my No-More-Dark-Spots Oats and my Powerhouse Quinoa breakfast dishes, my Stress-Fighting Salmon Cakes lunch recipe, my Revitalizing Goji Greatness snack, and my Omega-3 Garlic Barramundi with Mushrooms & Wild Rice dinner, to name a few. Naturally, oats, quinoa and wild rice can be beneficially incorporated into a diet adhering to The Young Skin Diet's principles even if my provided recipes are not specifically used.

As with oats and quinoa, other foods also provide antioxidants that impart anti-inflammation effects, and this is an important tool for fighting chronic low-level inflammation that ages skin.

Fourth, foods with antioxidants can impart anti-inflammatory effects since oxidative stress is responsible for chronic inflammation precipitating problems like psoriasis, dermatitis, rheumatoid arthritis and asthma.

A good example of this antioxidant/anti-inflammatory relationship is found in my Superantioxidant Allspice Mango recipe. Mangos are one of the only sources of mangiferin (a so-called "super-antioxidant"), which has been shown to combat oxidation, cancer, infection, allergy, pain and, yes, inflammation – all widespread benefits that support healthy, youthful skin.

Antioxidants can fight the precursors of inflammation.

Other antioxidant-rich, anti-inflammatory recipes include my Restorative Hot Honey Fruit (with capsaicin, a strong anti-inflammatory) and my Tone 'n Texture Shrimp 'n Veggies, which features the astaxanthin antioxidant/anti-inflammatory agent from shrimp and combines that agent with phytochemicals in red onions that are powerful anti-inflammatories.

These anti-inflammatory foods help soothe the body's systems back to normal function. They enable the body's natural processes to operate in such way as to promote healthy and beautiful skin. Ingredients included in my preferred recipes were selected in part for their antioxidant profiles and anti-inflammation effects. They can be incorporated into the diet to fight inflammation, even if the recipes I provide are not used.

As with meals, topical treatments that are part of The Young Skin Diet are designed to effectuate anti-inflammatory responses in the skin. Turmeric, for example, is a powerful anti-inflammatory and is accordingly a part of the treatment regimen. So are ginger, olive oil and honey, all of which appear in my given skin treatments.

Though all my recommended recipes and treatments exhibit beneficial anti-inflammation effects, a handful of specific foods and food combinations that are noteworthy in this regard are included in the following recipes:

- **Anti-Wrinkle Spiced Salmon & Asparagus:** Chinook, or king, salmon contains the highest levels of Omega-3 fatty acids among wild salmon varieties, providing more than 2,000 milligrams of total Omega-3's per 100 gram (a little less than 4 ounces) serving size. The overwhelming majority – more than 90% – of that Omega-3 fat is EPA and DHA, which are the most powerful anti-inflammatory Omega-3's available.

- **Rejuvenating Mykonos Mediterranean Salad:** Anchovies stored in extra virgin olive oil maintain their Omega-3 fatty acids better than when stored in other liquids like seed oils. Anchovies provide around 2,000 milligrams of EPA and DHA type Omega-3 fats per 100 grams of food. Kalamata olives called for in the recipe contain phenolics with powerful anti-inflammatory effects, and olive oil provides ALA Omega-3 fatty acids.
- **Anti-Oxidant Tropics Oats:** The beta-glucans from rolled oats exhibit powerful anti-inflammation effects, and chia seeds provide essential ALA Omega-3 fatty acids. In half an ounce of chia seeds, there are roughly 2,500 milligrams of ALA Omega-3 fats, which comprise about 75% of the food's total fat content – the chia seed's Omega-6 to Omega-3 ratio is about 0.33, helping promote achievement of a more balanced, inflammation-fighting overall Omega-6/Omega-3 fat ratio.
- **Restorative Hot Honey Fruit:** Capsaicin found in cayenne pepper exerts chemical effects at the cellular level to inhibit inflammation in the body.

The Young Skin Diet emphasizes anti-inflammatory foods so that nutrients can be efficiently and effectively delivered to skin to give it a youthful, healthy appearance.

3. Pro-collagen/Pro-elastin

Collagen and elastin are two important protein complexes found in the extracellular matrix in our dermis. Since this extracellular matrix of connective tissue can be thought of as the "glue" that gives our skin its dimensional structure and shape, as well as its flexibility and elasticity characteristics, the health and quantity of collagen and elastin in our skin have direct implications for our appearance.

Robust collagen and elastin are associated with youthful, smooth skin – healthy skin. When these protein complexes are depleted, however, we are left with sagging and wrinkled, damaged-looking skin that does not perform as it should.

It is relevant to note that the collagen and elastin populations in the body are dynamic, undergoing degradation over time and regeneration, with new proteins replacing the old. As we age and as our skin absorbs environmental damage as from UV exposure, three important components of the proteins' renewal process are altered.

Depleted collagen and elastin make skin appear aged.

First, the rate of degradation of the complexes increases. The population of collagen and elastin already in place declines because the rate at which it breaks down accelerates over time and under environmental duress. Second, the rate of generation of new protein complexes slows, so the availability of new collagen and elastin to replace the old declines. These two forces work in concert to profoundly affect the overall quantity and health of collagen and elastin in the skin since 1) the proteins' total populations decline and 2) their average "age" increases.

↑ RATE OF DECLINE + ↓ RATE OF RENEWAL = ↓ OVERALL QUANTITY &
HEALTH OF COLLAGEN & ELASTIN

The third component of the proteins' renewal process that is altered relates to the complex interplay of minerals, including silica and calcium, in the skin. Both silica and calcium have bearing on skin health since collagen and elastin are formed largely of silica and since calcium plays an important role in connection with keratin, a protein structure in the epidermis. However, in the event collagen or elastin is damaged, calcium can bind to them, causing cross-links that precipitate wrinkles and sagging. As we age, as we absorb environmental damage and as we consume imbalanced diets, our bodies may be unequipped with sufficient available silica to generate new connective skin proteins, or damaged skin proteins may be subjected to unwanted calcium deposition, or both.

Altogether, these forces working against the health of collagen and elastin in our skin press into stark relief the imperative that we consume a diet that promotes the health and new formation of these crucial tissues. The Young Skin Diet emphasizes five beneficial components of nutrition for pro-collagen/pro-elastin dieting as manifested in the lists of recommended foods and, most powerfully, in the provided recipes.

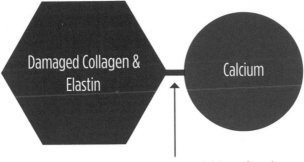

Bind = Cross-Linking + Wrinkles + Sagging

The first component relates to strategic antioxidant and anti-inflammatory consumption.

Both antioxidants and anti-inflammatories are beneficial for collagen and elastin since they blunt the damage-related processes that can accelerate degradation of the proteins and inhibit new protein formation.

Beta-carotene, for instance, which is the plant-derived form of the vitamin A antioxidant most readily assimilated into the human body, has been shown to enhance collagen production, improve skin elasticity and resolve facial wrinkles.

Beta-carotene's antioxidant benefits are magnified in combination with tochoperhols including vitamin E. Accordingly, recipes like my Age-Defying Tropical Fruit Dessert combine beta-carotene sources cantaloupe and honeydew with tocopherol-rich pumpkin seeds, as an example of pro-collagen strategic combination.

Vitamin A and vitamin E are powerful pro-collagen inputs.

The other antioxidants and anti-inflammatories described in detail in earlier sections of this book confer similar benefits, and other strategic combinations are detailed in my provided recipes.

Consumption of certain vitamins, for reasons other than their antioxidant and anti-inflammation effects, is the second component of The Young Skin Diet's pro-collagen/pro-elastin focus.

Certain vitamins in addition to antioxidant vitamins A and E have been individually identified as particularly beneficial for collagen and elastin health.

Although it is certainly the case that sufficient and balanced food-based sourcing of all vitamins is critical for optimal skin health, **some individual vita-**

mins are emphasized in The Young Skin Diet because they are particularly relevant in keeping our skin healthy and young by supporting the body's connective tissues.

Vitamin C, for example, supports the biological processes that synthesize collagen in the body. Among recipes in The Young Skin Diet that are excellent sources of vitamin C is my Procollagen Sweet Potato & Eggs. This meal also provides the body with a dose of lysine and proline amino acids. This is beneficial since, when combined, **vitamin C binds with lysine and proline to form procollagen, which the body uses directly in the manufacture of collagen.**

Vitamin K2 has been identified as especially important in "directing" allocation of calcium in the body so that it is placed in beneficial locations like the bones and not in soft tissue. Research continues to evaluate the role of vitamin K2 and its connection with calcium deposition outside of bone and cardiovascular health. However, the existing research surrounding vitamin K2 suggests myriad benefits for overall health, and its method of action for directing calcium to appropriate uses is suggestive of a positive role in the skin by **helping minimize likelihood that unwanted calcifications of the collagen and elastin protein complexes occurs.**

Coupled with the fact that most Western diets are quite low in vitamin K2, consumption of foods containing the vitamin is recommended as part of the overall plan for eating for young skin. Accordingly, eggs (particularly egg yolks), which are a good source of vitamin K2 among other things, are found in various recipes of The Young Skin Diet, including Make-Your-Skin Glow Spinach & Eggs and Natural Sunscreen Green Eggs & Omegas.

By eating a diet of varied whole foods encompassing those listed in my provided food lists and/or included in the recipes set forth in this book, pro-collagen/pro-elastin vitamins will be sufficiently consumed for young skin.

Similar to vitamins, dietary minerals play an important role in collagen and elastin health and are thus the third component of the pro-collagen/pro-elastin focus of The Young Skin Diet.

Sufficient intake of minerals that may often be lacking in modern Western diets, including silica, choline, manganese, magnesium and iron, is important for the health of collagen, elastin and the extracellular matrix in the skin.

As with vitamins, sufficient food-based sourcing of all dietary minerals is crucial for skin health and appearance since any deficiencies will harm the biological processes underlying great skin. A varied diet emphasizing plant-based, unprocessed, whole foods imparts proper mineral allowances and supports these operations. Certain specific minerals nevertheless warrant mention here because of their particular importance to skin's collagen, elastin and extracellular matrix.

Silica is a main component of the collagen and elastin protein complexes. It is accordingly the case that, **when silica levels are insufficient, new collagen and elastin synthesis is constrained**, adding to the depletion and aging of those proteins in the body. In this vein, the addition of bioavailable silica to the diet has been demonstrated to confer positive cosmetic results on photodamaged skin.

While silica is one of the most abundant elements on the planet and found in virtually all vegetables, **the bioavailability of silica can differ materially from source to source.** Bioavailiability refers to the body's rate of absorption of the mineral from food. Among the best sources are green beans, exhibiting an estimated 44% absorption rate.

Choline and manganese also play parts in the complex mineral dance that leads to collagen synthesis. These minerals, from highly bioaccessible sources like green beans, chickpeas, cucumber and zucchini are found throughout recipes in The Young Skin Diet, such as my Smooth Skin Zucchini with Chicken, Strong Skin Spinach & Chickpeas, and my Tighten-Your-Skin Slow Cooker Yellow Curry, to name a few examples of strategic pro-collagen/pro-elastin food selections.

Magnesium has been linked with the body's production of hyaluronic acid, a component of the extracellular matrix where collagen and elastin reside. **The hyaluronic acid molecule is most abundant in tissues like skin (where roughly 50% of the body's stores reside) and helps tissues retain moisture and volume, essentially "plumping" areas where it is most densely clustered.** It is for this reason that hyaluronic acid features in various cosmetic, anti-aging and "dermal filler" products. The body's stores of hyaluronic acid decline over time, which leads to aged appearance markers like sagging and wrinkled skin. What's more, with declining concentrations of hyaluronic acid, the effects of any reductions in collagen and elastin levels are magnified. Hyaluronic acid, collagen and elastin work together to keep skin young looking.

By ensuring sufficient magnesium in the diet, the body's natural production of hyaluronic acid is promoted and loss of the molecule from the extracellular matrix is blunted. Dark, leafy greens like spinach and seeds like those from pumpkins are particularly good food sources of magnesium, while some legumes like **chickpeas can provide hyaluronic acid directly.** Recipes such as my Strong Skin Spinach & Chickpeas and my Age-Defying Tropical Fruit Dessert provide these ingredients in beneficial, strategic combinations and preparations.

Though The Young Skin Diet emphasizes plant-based foods, one particularly important pro-collagen/pro-elastin dietary input can be found only in meats. **This input, carnosine, is accordingly prioritized in The Young Skin Diet and forms the fourth component of The Young Skin Diet's pro-collagen/pro-elastin strategy.**

The carnosine dipeptide, found in meats, is vital in warding off oxidative damage, AGE production and cross-linking in the skin's intracellular matrix that lead to wrinkling and sagging.

Carnosine has been shown to have significant radical scavenging activity against the most harmful hydroxyl radical oxidative agents in the body. The peptide also exhibits pro-health effects associated with resolving protein damage in the body (including in protein structures collagen and elastin), as well as forestalling cross-linking, AGE production and inflammation.

Carnosine's youth-promoting activities are varied and potent.

Richest in red meats and poultry, carnosine also is found in lower concentrations in some fish, eggs and other animal-based foods. Poultry's carnosine concentration is second to red meats, carrying levels roughly one-third that of leaner cuts of red meat. However, chicken also carries a significantly lower risk level of negative health and skin impacts associated with red meat's other nutritional components. For this reason, and because of the variety of culinary applications and cooking (including "wet" cooking) techniques applicable to poultry like chicken, chicken is the preferred source of carnosine in The Young Skin Diet.

A handful of chicken-based dishes appear in The Young Skin Diet's provided recipes for these reasons, including my Tighten-Your-Skin Slow Cooker Yellow Curry and my Smooth Skin Zucchini with Chicken.

Chicken, as it turns out, also provides amino acids that are critical for collagen and elastin support. **Balanced amino acid intake is the fifth and final part of The Young Skin Diet's strategy for pro-collagen/pro-elastin dieting.**

A diet rich in balanced essential amino acids is crucial for maintaining a biological state supportive of collagen and elastin maintenance.

Essential amino acids are those components of proteins that we must derive from our diet; we can't manufacture essential amino acids ourselves.

Because collagen and elastin are proteins manufactured from amino acids, it is imperative that we have sufficient levels of these building blocks to support collagen and elastin synthesis, and that we consistently provide our body useful amino acids so that we don't stress our system. **In states of insufficient amino acids, collagen and elastin synthesis in the skin may not occur because the building blocks are unavailable or needed elsewhere in the body.** Amino acid shortages can age skin.

Consuming the right amount and composition of amino acids implies eating sufficient levels of highly bioavailable protein from a variety of sources with regularity though the day. The Young Skin Diet's recipes are engineered to provide good amino acid profiles from highly bioaccessible protein. Chicken, as mentioned, is one excellent contributor of amino acids. Also included among the recipes that are great sources of complete amino acids are my Photoaging Protection Quinoa & Vegetable Poached Eggs, Powerhouse Quinoa, and Skin-Strengthening Veggie Egg Scramble.

In addition to these nutritional components of The Young Skin Diet, treatments applied externally have been shown to enhance skin's collagen population, skin elasticity, skin resilience and capillary action.

A dampened warm towel compress, as used in my No-More-Irritation Cucumber Treatment, for example, has been shown to increase skin elasticity and improve blood circulation in capillaries feeding the skin. Coconut oil, a part of my Skin-Brightening Coconut Oil Exfoliant treatment, is associated with significant improvements in skin elasticity. And the combination of lemon juice and cane sugar, included in two of my treatments, provides two alpha-hydroxy acids (citric acid and glycolic acid) that work directly against collagen loss and support improved collagen populations in the skin.

Though all my recommended recipes and treatments exhibit beneficial pro-collagen/pro-elastin effects, a handful of specific foods and food combinations with such benefits that are noteworthy include the following:

- **Smooth Skin Zucchini with Chicken:** The carnosine in chicken and phytochemicals (including allicin) in garlic fight AGE formation, cross-linking and collagen degradation using two complementary pathways. Zucchini's manganese enables the body to use choline found in chicken in collagen formation.

- **Hydrating Cucumber and Watermelon Cooldown:** Like green beans, cucumber provides highly bioaccessible silica, which is the primary building block of the body's connective tissues, including collagen and elastin.
- **Repair-Your-Skin Thai Quinoa & Kale Salad:** Quinoa's complete amino acid profile helps ensure sufficient availability of protein components for collagen and elastin synthesis. The vitamin C from lime helps the body absorb iron from kale, which effect is important because of iron's role in supporting collagen production.
- **Healthy Skin Pistachio-Melon-Cherry Panache:** Pistachios and watermelon use two different biochemical pathways to improve circulatory function, including capillary function feeding the skin. Cherry's anthocyanin antioxidants have demonstrated anti-inflammation effects that promote metabolic efficiency and thus help healthy skin cells benefit from added circulatory throughput that can shuttle collagen- and elastin-building nutrients to the critical areas of the skin.

The Young Skin Diet calls for consumption of foods that are collagen and elastin boosting to give skin youthful flexibility and elasticity.

4. Pro-hydration

Hydration. Water. Moisture. Whatever we call it, it's needed for a healthy body and beautiful skin. Good hydration helps the body to flush unwanted waste from the system and supports all the body's processes. A primary defense against dry, brittle skin is water.

For skin, it is relevant to focus on both internal hydration and external moisturizing. Internal hydration directly supports the skin's metabolic function, while external moisturizing practices help keep moisture dissipation from the skin's surface low, so dryness is minimized, which maintains protection against wrinkling and promotes exfoliation.

Internal hydration depends primarily upon sufficient water intake. The "optimal" amount of water consumption varies by individual on the basis of such factors as body mass, activity level and the prevailing climate of habitation. However, a general point of guidance that can be used as a starting point in fine-tuning our water consumption for young skin is about 64 ounces per day.

As important as water quantity is, so too is the timing of consumption. Imbibing water first thing in the morning is crucial since the body tends to be parched after a night's sleep. Consistent water drinking throughout the day helps keep the body's systems functioning efficiently. And taking water with food can aid digestion and the absorption of nutrients. All this supports young skin since consistency of moisture availability is key in keeping skin healthy and hydrated.

In connection with taking water with food, **we often overlook the importance of consuming foods that are themselves good sources of hydration.** Fruits and vegetables are comprised largely of water and, as with most of the components of whole plant foods, that water plays a role in assisting the body's utilization of the plants' vitamins and other nutrients. Many recipes in The Young Skin Diet emphasize the hydrating power of plant foods, and virtually all contain whole foods that impart moisture. My Collagen-Boosting Strawberry-Melon Refresh and Hydrating Cucumber & Watermelon Cooldown recipes are some of my favorites for hydration. My recommended foods generally help ensure good hydration, so long as they are consumed with variety and balance.

An element of The Young Skin Diet that resides somewhere in between water and hydrating foods is tea, which offers a bevy of antioxidants and other benefits along with flavorful and non-caloric hydration. Homemade tea recipes like my Restorative Ginger & Honey Tea are engineered to combat infection and microbial presence, thereby reducing skin inflammation and redness, but they also provide several ounces of water in a serving. As part of The Young Skin Diet, consuming tea is highly recommended as a daily young-skin habit.

External hydration is likewise important for skin since excessive dryness can lead to premature wrinkling, inflammation and inefficient exfoliation (which itself can result in blemishes and dullness). The skin treatments in my program are designed to enhance moisture levels in skin by servicing those cells dependent upon osmotic processes for hydration, by exfoliating old and damaged skin cells efficiently and by calming inflammation that can be brought on by excessive dryness.

For example, coconut oil in my Skin Brightening Coconut Oil Exfoliant treatment has been shown to significantly enhance skin moisture and elasticity. **Topical application of coconut oil has been linked with hydration and elasticity levels 140% and 175% of untreated skin**, respectively, if used regularly for 3 weeks, and skin treated with coconut oil exhibits more than 3 times the elasticity gain of skin treated with lotions absent coconut oil's fats and chemicals.

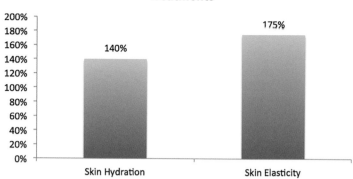

Percent Improvement Using TYSD Natural Skin Treatments

Honey and olive oil in combination are similarly noted for resolving dryness, maintaining skin hydration and enhancing skin elasticity, even among individuals with dermatitis/eczema and psoriasis. This powerful combination is used my No-More-Inflammation Honey & Olive Oil Mask.

And the alpha-hydroxy acids derived from lemon juice and cane sugar act as chemexfoliants to remove old and desiccated skin from the epidermal surface, revealing newer and better hydrated cells. These ingredients are called for in my Lemon Water & Cane Sugar Skin Toning Mask and work to reveal younger looking skin.

In addition to these internal and external hydrating focuses, there is another element of "pro-hydration" that forms a core part of The Young Skin Diet. This pro-hydration element relates to the use of "wet" cooking techniques to heat food since wet (and thus lower-temperature) cooking practices produce far fewer advanced glycation end products than traditional Western "dry" cooking conventions.

Since AGEs are believed substantially responsible for a host of health maladies, including premature aging in the skin, reducing them is an important part of The Young Skin Diet. In general, wet cooking techniques include boiling, poaching, blanching, steaming, cooking in stews and preparing foods in slow cookers. Dry cooking techniques (which rely upon higher temperatures) are those like grilling, baking, broiling, frying and roasting.

Many recipes in The Young Skin Diet rely upon wet cooking techniques to take advantage of the benefits of reducing AGEs in the diet. Those recipes that rely upon dry cooking techniques utilize herbs, spices, citrus juices or vinegars to protect foods during cooking to reduce AGE production. Even if none of the recipes provided in this book is used, attention should always be paid to food preparation techniques since they often are as important as the foods themselves in ensuring good nutrition and skin outcomes. Low-heat and "wet" cooking should be used whenever possible. And the use of marinades and spices should always be incorporated if dry cooking is necessitated. I recommend perusing the recipes included in the back of this book for examples of wet cooking techniques, appropriate marinating practices and advantageous spice mixes that keep AGE values low.

Notwithstanding the general recommendation for wet cooking, some foods are less prone to AGE formation and, in fact, the research indicates substantial health benefits from a particular dry preparation method for certain of those foods – as, for example, in my recommendation of cooking tomato in olive oil on the skillet in my Make-Your-Skin-Glow Spinach and Eggs. This combination and preparation approach is linked with at least 20% higher availability of tomatoes' lycopene for the skin.

Though all my recommended recipes and treatments are engineered for pro-hydration benefits, a handful of specific foods and food combinations that are noteworthy in this connection include the following:

- **Natural Sunscreen Green Eggs & Omegas:** With poaching rather than frying, the AGE formation in foods, particularly meats and other animal products like eggs, is minimized. Eggs' myriad health benefits for skin, including hydrating Omega-3 fatty acids, remain intact with "wet" cooking techniques but can be destroyed with high-temperature "dry" cooking methods like frying.
- **Age-Defying Tropical Fruit Dessert:** Cantaloupe and honeydew both are comprised mostly of water by mass, so their pro-hydration effects begin with their moisture content. Their high potassium content complements the high potassium level of pumpkin seeds to help correct any sodium-potassium imbalances that can lead to dehydration.
- **Skin-Plumping Berry Smoothie:** In addition to the natural hydrating power of berries and citrus, banana peel helps support healthy and hydrated skin by providing antifungal and antibiotic phytochemicals that improve skin resilience and thus help reduce moisture loss.

The Young Skin Diet hydrates the skin to keep toxins flushed out of the system and to keep skin looking plump and moisturized.

5. Anti-stress

There are two chief strains of stress that bear down on us, seemingly without reprieve. **The first is environmental stress – UV rays, automobile exhaust, cigarette smoke, pesticide residue on foods, chemicals leeched from plastics, mold, antibiotics in meats and hundreds of other, similar things that force our bodies to allocate resources to warding off their ill effects.** Which, in the aggregate, can leave our bodies woefully out of balance.

Many of these environmental stressors, particularly UV rays, pesticide residue, chemicals and antibiotics, The Young Skin Diet is engineered to directly combat or minimize. In the case of UV rays, for example, The Young Skin Diet emphasizes foods rich in antioxidants and anti-inflammatories that protect cells from damage and help repair past harms. Foods proven to directly enhance UV resistance or correct UV damage, like green tea, pomegranate seeds, and combinations of avocado and tomato, to name a few, are called upon regularly as strategic selections in The Young Skin Diet.

Regarding pesticides, chemicals and antibiotics from our foods, The Young Skin Diet eschews processed goods typically subjected to harsh pesticides and chemicals, and it prioritizes organic produce and certain types of fish that minimize our exposure to pesticides, chemicals and un-prescribed antibiotics. Meanwhile, red meats and pork, which often are raised with antibiotic regimens, are left out altogether.

See my recommended foods lists for "do" and "don't" foods in this regard, and see the provided recipes, which pages summarize the science regarding UV-fighting foods, for more information on ingredients that combat UV damage.

A NOTE ABOUT ORGANIC PRODUCE

A 2015 study conducted by the Swedish Environmental Research Institute followed a family of 5 for a 2-week period while the parents and children first consumed all conventional produce for one week followed by one week of all organic produce. During the period studied, pesticide levels in the family members decreased on average by a factor greater than 9, with an even higher reduction factor for the children (close to 12), when conventional produce was replaced with organic varieties. On the basis of such research, organic foods are recommended as part of The Young Skin Diet. The presence of pesticides and other chemicals in the body can harm skin and overall health.

Other environmental stressors, such as car fumes and secondhand smoke, are naturally best if avoided. But modern life makes absolute avoidance impracticable. Nevertheless, **antioxidants garnered from a broad array of plant-based foods have been shown to help protect DNA and bodily tissues like skin from the damage brought on by such stressors.** Since a cornerstone of The Young Skin Diet is varied plant foods, these stressors are addressed as well.

The second type of stressor (i.e., not environmental) that afflicts us is psychological or emotional in nature. This is "internal" stress that, yes, may be precipitated by outside factors (like heavy traffic or a meddlesome coworker) but which principally manifests inside us. Unlike environmental stressors like UV rays that "fry" our skin directly, internal stressors work more subtly – more insidiously – to undermine our health and the youthfulness of our skin.

↑ ENVIRONMENTAL STRESS + ↑ PSYCHOLOGICAL STRESS = ↓ SKIN HEALTH & YOUTHFULNESS

Prolonged internal stress can limit the efficiency of our digestive processes, thereby impeding our ability to extract nutrition from the foods we eat and thus harming our bodies and skin.

Abiding stress can cause elevated blood pressure, which renders our circulatory system – the delivery system for our life-sustaining and skin-maintaining inputs – less efficient and places untenable demands on organs like our heart, brain and skin.

And **sustained emotional stress causes imbalances in hormone levels, resulting in chronically high levels of cortisol (the "stress hormone"), which can directly harm the skin by accelerating degradation of collagen, impeding wound healing and dehydrating us.** Sustained high levels of cortisol also cause a bunch of other nasty health problems that indirectly affect our skin and appearance, like harming muscle synthesis.

So managing our internal stress is crucial for great health and youthful looking skin. But how can we use foods to keep our internal stress in check, our systems working efficiently and our cortisol levels down?

The Young Skin Diet depends upon three anti-stress pillars for great-skin stress relief.

The first is the consumption (or avoidance) of foods with salutary (or deleterious) consequences for our body's management of emotional stress and the cortisol hormone linked with stress.

Foods can directly affect emotional stress levels.

Among the most studied and interesting of foods with serious anti-stress credentials are teas. Rooibos tea, for instance, boasts a raft of health benefits, including the provision of a unique antioxidant profile, but it also has been shown to have a powerful calming effect on various pathways in the body's nervous system and to play a role in the downregulation of cortisol.

Other teas, including black tea and green tea as well as herbal teas, have exhibited similar anti-stress benefits. Such teas are accordingly part of The Young Skin Diet for their antioxidant benefits, hormone-balancing effects and, also linked with stress, their digestion-aiding properties.

Foods high in Omega-3 fats have been shown to ameliorate stress, while foods packing lots of Omega-6 fats have contrary effects. The Young Skin Diet therefore calls for inclusion of Omega-3 rich foods like salmon, anchovies, barramundi and eggs from hens fed diets that are rich in Omega-3s.

Whole fruits and vegetables, and strategic combinations of them in particular, also fight stress. Cherries and bananas work synergistically to promote sleep and feelings of well-being, thus enabling restorative rest, reprieve from stress and reductions in cortisol. Cherries and bananas both contain serotonin, a sleep-assisting agent and mood booster. Bananas also contain tryptophan, and cherries provide melatonin, both of which promote natural sleep. Bananas and cherries are combined in my Sweet Deams Smoothie.

Just as certain foods reduce stress and counteract cortisol production, foods high in refined carbohydrates, simple sugars without accompanying fiber, and alcohol can wreak havoc on the body's hormonal stability and result in higher stress levels. So, these sorts of foods are absent from The Young Skin Diet.

The second anti-stress pillar that is part of The Young Skin Diet comes from what I like to call the "zen of cooking." It is well established that psychological stress can be reduced through a variety of avocations like undertaking exercise, listening to or playing music, breathing deeply, pursuing mindfulness, practicing gratefulness and tending to hobbies. A large part of these activities' ability to reduce stress is found in their requirement that, in order to fully pursue them, we must let go of the rush of the day (or whatever is causing us stress), pause to set our minds to a new purpose and focus on something that, with effort and attention, we can succeed at doing.

The conditions that cause avocations like playing music to reduce stress are also present in cooking.

When cooking, attention is required (lest there be a kitchen fire), and there is the opportunity to indulge the senses with aromas, palate-pleasing flavors and beautiful presentation. Moreover, we can achieve success and completion through our efforts, particularly given the ease and simplicity of The Young Skin Diet's recipes and recommended foods. **Thus, the recipes that are part of this book have twofold benefits on our skin: first, through their nutrition; and second, through the act of guiding our attention to something new that presents the mind an opportunity to learn and focus on the act of preparation.**

It has accordingly been my endeavor to not only create nutritionally optimized recipes that follow guidance from my research on youthful skin but to help foster a sense of calmness and anti-stress in connection with the recipes' preparation. Pictures accompanying The Young Skin Diet's dishes are meant to look beautiful and uncomplicated so as to add to the serenity in your life and provide a place of escape from life's stressors as you complete the steps to turn the recipes into healthy meals that taste great and restore your skin.

The photos also serve a functional purpose by illustrating what finished products from the kitchen look like and/or by demonstrating the simplicity of ingredients. These recipes are not stress-inducing; rather, they're easy and simple and, as with any stress-defeating avocation, richly reward your efforts.

The third anti-stress pillar relates to the skin treatments outlined as part of The Young Skin Diet. How do these deflate stress? In part, simply because they're fun! When was the last time you were given permission – even encouraged – to smear honey, lemon juice or coconut oil all over your face? There is something fundamentally gratifying and de-stressing about the act of doing so, even if peer-reviewed research hasn't yet addressed the benefits of the act, focusing instead on the benefits of the act simply having been done.

Perhaps more importantly, the treatments that are part of The Young Skin Diet typically involve leaving the mask in place for about 10 minutes. So these treatments give you a built-in window of "me-time" for reflection, deep breathing and quiet solitude, which can help defuse even the most stressful days. (It can also be a great time to enjoy an extra cup of anti-stress tea.)

Skin treatments outlined in The Young Skin Diet fight stress in two ways.

As with meal and snack recipes found in The Young Skin Diet, the treatments serve a dual role in combating the ill effects of stress on our skin. They first counteract some of the negative consequences of chronic stress like the accelerated degradation of collagen by presenting pro-collagen alpha-hydroxy acids and anti-inflammatories to the epidermis. And they second help stop stress at its source by providing a good-for-you excuse for respite and quiet and a break from the outside world.

Though all my recommended recipes and treatments are engineered for anti-stress benefits, a handful of specific foods and food combinations that are noteworthy in this connection are included in the following recipes:

- **Stress-Fighting Salmon Cakes:** Canned salmon contains as much Omega-3 fatty acid content as fresh or frozen salmon fillets, thus imparting powerful anti-stress benefits associated with Omega-3 fats. In addition, the capsaicin found in pepper sauce is a natural analgesic that combats pain. Since cortisol levels spike in the presence of physical pain, and since sleep can be interrupted by pain (which also raises cortisol production), capsaicin is powerfully anti-stress.
- **No-More-Dark-Spots Oats:** Among other beneficial ingredients, pomegranate seeds, which contain ellagic acid, protect skin from UV stress. Walnuts have been found beneficial in enhancing the body's resilience to the onset of diseases associated with systemic stress. And chia seeds provide anti-stress Omega-3 fats.
- **Stress Relief Black Tea with Lemon:** As with other teas, consumption of black tea causes reductions in cortisol levels in the body. Interestingly, the consumption of black tea also has been linked to greater subjective

scores in relaxation. **Since the cortisol stress pathway can both cause and be caused by reduced relaxation, black tea's effects on stress appear to be dual-sided and thus very powerful.**

The Young Skin Diet is engineered to combat both environmental and emotional stress to keep skin looking vibrant and youthful.

6. Non-allergenic

Allergens are curious things. They would be totally innocuous to the body if not for the fact that they trigger an immune system response. Nevertheless, the immune system's reaction to the presence of allergens does occur. And it sets off a cascade of troublesome symptoms in people that can show up in the body's internal processes and the skin, leading to effects that damage the skin's tissues.

Swelling, redness, itchiness and even more damaging body responses manifest sometimes rapidly and last for a long while following allergenic exposure. **In connection with our skin, allergens are problematic because we may not be aware that certain foods – often staples in the traditional Western diet – trigger mild allergic reactions in us.** And those reactions, which can be essentially chronic, slowly degrade the evenness and smoothness – the attractiveness – of our skin.

To account for this, The Young Skin Diet culls out the most common food allergens that:

1. do not provide significant skin or health benefits;
2. may provide skin or health benefits, but which benefits can be readily found in non-allergenic foods; or
3. may provide skin or health benefits, but which benefits are still outweighed by the foods' potential harms.

This means there is no wheat, no gluten, no dairy, no casein, no soy, no corn and no peanuts in The Young Skin Diet.

Because the foods that do support great skin are of such great variety and so tasty when prepared properly, these allergenic foods, staples of the typical Western diet though they may be, are not essential to good flavor, enjoyable eating or young skin.

These seven common allergens may not be problematic for every person. It is nevertheless the case that, from my analysis of nutrition research, from my conversations with many people who suffer from diagnosed food allergies, and from my personal experience with food allergens, it appears that some of us may have mild allergenic responses to certain of these foods and simply not know it.

Indeed, **one study (among many, similar studies with similar results) evaluated pediatric patients with severe atopic dermatitis and found that more than half of those patients exhibited food sensitivities.** It further found that removing the allergenic foods from patients' diets improved their dermatitis significantly relative to patients without diet alterations.

With an appropriately balanced diet of foods recommended as part of The Young Skin Diet, **the body does not need any of these possibly allergenic foods.** Since they may be problematic and are not essential, there is little risk in removing these foods from our diet, but there is significant potential upside.

By eliminating these foods, we give our immune systems a chance to calm down and we give our bodies a chance to relax and refocus attention on processes that support healthy looking skin. Puffiness, redness and itchiness – things some people simply believe are an intrinsic part of their complexions – are given opportunity to resolve themselves and yield healthy, great-looking skin.

It is worth sharing here my own experience with food allergens since that experience was eye opening to me about the power of food sensitivities. Several years ago, my husband underwent an abrupt and dramatic change in his health. A lifelong athlete and fitness enthusiast, my husband was the picture of robust health. Then, he suddenly became ill with symptoms that included severe abdominal pain, dramatic weight loss and lethargy. The rapidity of change in his health was shocking. In just weeks, he had gone from active to listless. Upbeat to depressed. Muscular to skeletal. My husband underwent months of testing, scans and consultations. The mysterious cause of his illness remained unexplained, and his condition continued to deteriorate.

It was only at the urging of a friend who knew our desperation that my husband (and I, for support) undertook a systematic elimination diet. Slowly, my husband's problems with gluten, dairy and peanuts were revealed. Much less quickly than his health had diminished, his energy, upbeat personality and athletic build returned. Common food allergens stayed out of his diet, and remain absent from his diet now, years later.

My husband's health experience was enough to convince me of the power of food allergens, and how **allergies can both hide from view and worsen unexpectedly.** However, even more convincing was my own response to removing common food allergens from my diet.

I'd only stopped eating certain foods to make my husband's elimination diet easier on him. I wasn't like I had any food allergies. I could eat anything I wanted without worry…right? Well, as it turns out, I should have been a bit more worried. Within several weeks of culling certain common food allergens from my diet, I had more energy, easier digestion and, yes, clearer and more evenly toned skin. **This pattern of unrecognized food allergies is not unique to me but is reflected in various studies** like the pediatric study mentioned earlier.

Since they're not necessary, can be a problem, and do not have sufficiently strong pro-skin arguments in their favor, wheat, gluten, dairy, casein, soy, corn and peanuts are not part of The Young Skin Diet.

The Young Skin Diet eliminates common food allergens to keep skin calm and healthy.

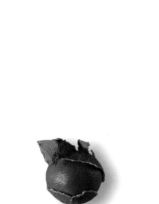

These themes – The Six Principles of the Young Skin Diet – form the backbone of my program for rejuvenated, healthy skin. They all derive from a wealth of scientific evidence. And these six principles are most fully and directly put to action in my provided meal plans and recipes, though they also can be implemented via adoption of the general food selection, combination and preparation strategies set forth in my recipes, food lists and everyday habits list. **In this regard, every recipe in this book has been designed to maximize anti-oxidation, anti-inflammation, pro-collagen/pro-elastin, pro-hydration and anti-stress effects in the body, and to be non-allergenic.**

As a practical matter, how is this done?

First, by using only those categories of foods that benefit the body, and by avoiding those that don't.

Vegetables, fruits, cold water fish, seeds, and sources of healthy fats and proteins are found in my recommended foods list and recipes, while processed ingredients, added refined sugars, preservatives, excess salt, red meats, simple carbohydrates and common allergens are not. It's just that simple.

For those skeptical that anything good (or good tasting) could come of a diet bereft of lots of refined sugars and simple carbs, I encourage giving the recipes and recommended foods a try – let their flavors and results speak for themselves.

Part of using foods to benefit the body implies a high level of variety in what we eat. Which, from a culinary perspective, means a bounty of varied flavors, textures and exciting combinations. **Optimizing our diets for healthfulness and great skin means eating not just a select few good foods, but a wide range of good foods.** Doing so helps ensure that healthy food doesn't have to taste like "health food," and it helps ensure the additive, synergistic and cumulative benefits of eating a collection of young-skin foods are maximized.

Second, by researching each recommended food category to ensure that any recommended specific food in that category offers strong benefits with minimized (if any) downsides.

The "good" foods categories and "bad" foods categories are the simple part. However, there are some foods within "good" categories that, if not consumed carefully, can cause undesirable results.

The spice nutmeg, for instance, like most other spices, is a great source of antioxidants and anti-inflammatories. Indeed, nutmeg contains powerful antioxidants including malabricone C and others which exhibit strong free radical scavenging activity and are useful as part of The Young Skin Diet. If too much nutmeg is consumed, though, the spice can cause both visual and auditory hallucinations similar to those associated with psychotropic drugs. Nutmeg, cloves and other spices with similar profiles are accordingly recommended to be used in moderation and are used appropriately and strategically (i.e., in beneficially synergistic combinations) in my provided recipes.

Certain fish, such as some types of mackerel, are among the greatest bearers of Omega-3 fatty acids and are thus highly nutritious for young skin. Unfortunately, many types of mackerel, like Spanish mackerel, are also very high in mercury content, which can poison the body. To avoid the prospect of harmful confusion, mackerel is simply left off the list of recommended fish and does not feature in any of my provided recipes.

My recipes rely upon well-understood and well-researched foods and upon healthy quantities of those foods – so the good is maximized and the bad is avoided.

Moreover, my research has helped me incorporate "best of breed" foods into my recipes and recommended food lists. For example, carnosine, which is found in meat, has been shown to reduce protein cross-linking in the skin and thus ward off wrinkles and other signs of aging. Among meats, poultry is the best source of carnosine because of its relatively low saturated fat content, ability to be readily prepared using wet cooking methods, and better overall healthiness profile compared with red meats and pork.

Teas, too, exhibit differences in nutrition impact. Home-brewed green teas and rooibos teas are particularly beneficial, while store-bought canned or bottled teas are not. Indeed, the catechins found in green tea, which can counteract oxidative stress and signs of aging, can be overwhelmingly degraded by processing and storage conditions.

Something else I've found in my research that helps maximize good and avoid bad is what I call "flavorful food synergy." This means that many foods that taste good together are actually better for you when consumed together. That's culinary common sense, and it comprises the next part of my principles in action.

Third, by engineering recipes to include foods that exhibit pro-health synergies with one another.

For example, tomatoes and broccoli exhibit stronger health benefits when coupled. Broccoli is rich in a flavonol called quercetin, which boasts powerful antioxidant and anti-inflammatory properties. The lycopene carotenoid in tomatoes can reduce the effects of UV photodamage in skin. Combined, the effects of broccoli and tomato are intensified. Plus, when tomatoes are cooked in olive oil, their lycopene molecules restructure to become more easily transmitted to skin tissue. My Skin-Strengthening Veggie Egg Scramble takes advantage of this synergy by combining broccoli, tomato and olive oil in an easy-to-make, tasty, healthy dish. These ingredients are, after all, staples of the Mediterranean diet.

Black pepper and turmeric exhibit synergistic properties as well. Curcumin and curcuminoids boast potent anti-inflammatory and pro-metabolic benefits and have been shown to interact with collagen to enhance dermal repair and reduce scarring. The piperine in black pepper enhances the bioavailiability of curcumin by 2,000%, making the combo one powerful synergistic pairing for skin health. To experience the benefits firsthand, I recommend giving my Tighten-Your-Skin Slow Cooker Yellow Curry a try. Flavorful? Absolutely: turmeric and black pepper are the primary constituents of yellow curry powder.

My research has similarly uncovered that varieties of citrus fruits, when consumed together, produce health synergies. My UV Protection Citrus Salad, for instance, combines orange and grapefruit to magnify their natural UV damage prevention. The flavor argument here is best made experientially: give mixed citrus a try.

I also found that citrus fruits help the body absorb nutrition from certain herbs and greens, which is why my Omega-3 Garlic Barramundi with Mushrooms & Wild Rice includes lemon and rosemary. The citrus flavonoids from lemon and polyphenols and diterpenes from rosemary have been shown to produce synergistic effects in protecting the epidermis from photoaging, improving resistance to damage by as much as 56%, and this flavor mix complements meats and fish wonderfully.

Similarly, eggs help usher plants' antioxidants into the body. My Photoaging Protection Quinoa & Vegetable Poached Eggs, Make-Your-Skin-Glow Spinach & Eggs and "Build Your Own Combination" spring lettuce and poached egg salad take advantage of the powerful benefits associated with combining vegetables and eggs. While many in the U.S. may not be accustomed to combining egg with vegetables, the practice is commonplace in traditional European eating, including Mediterranean eating, which has been empirically linked with good skin and aging outcomes.

Teas, too, benefit from a squeeze of lemon. Potent antioxidants in green tea known as catechins counteract oxidative stress and the signs of aging on skin. Lemon juice and its high levels of vitamin C protect catechins in the body from degradation and enable 500% greater absorption. Accordingly, many of my Morning Beverages are comprised of freshly-brewed tea with fresh-squeezed lemon or lime juice. The combination of tea with lemon is not merely healthy, but also tasty: it's no coincidence the combo is a favorite among tea drinkers.

And science tells us that some spices, like rosemary and other "green" herbs as well as vinegars and citrus juices, help stabilize foods when they're cooked. My Elasticity Boost Asian Fusion Salad, for example, relies upon rosemary to stabilize chicken while it sautés and prevent excessive formation of AGEs. The right spices and marinades enhance meats' flavors beautifully.

So I developed recipes that incorporate special relationships like these to help make every ingredient work as hard for skin health as possible. Fortuitously, many of these super-food combinations also taste fantastic – these are the "flavorful food synergies" I love so much.

The general takeaway from my research in this vein is that we eat our best when our meals incorporate many types of foods (especially foods from different food classes – e.g., combining fruits with vegetables, eggs with greens, etc.) and those foods are "whole" (i.e., unrefined, unprocessed and uncorrupted) since the macro- and micro-nutrient profiles of foods are most balanced and most likely to exhibit magnified benefits in these types of assemblage.

It is this latter general observation that means a varied diet comprising the foods encompassed by my recommended foods categories will yield synergistic benefits similar to those already delineated by science and incorporated into my recipes. For even more particular "flavorful food synergy" examples, I encourage review of the recipes included in this book, even if those recipes are not ultimately made as part of your adoption of The Young Skin Diet. This is because the recipes include scientific background on many powerful young-skin food combinations and can be used as inspiration for incorporating such combos into your everyday diet in dishes of your own creation. (I believe that when we have a deeper knowledge about foods, we make better choices and are energized to implement those choices regularly.)

Fourth, by developing recipes that use cooking techniques to enhance – or to protect – nutritional elements of foods.

Food is chemistry. When we prepare foods, we set off chemical cascades in ingredients. Some of these cascades enhance nutrition, while others degrade nutrition. My recipes rely on cooking techniques to protect or improve nutrition, not destroy it.

For instance, foods like tomatoes and carrots become richer in available nutrition when heated. Broccoli, on the other hand, is most nutritious when cooking times and temperatures are limited. Kale is best uncooked. Olive oil should not be subjected to too much heat, or else its good fats can be harmed.

All things equal, "wet" cooking techniques are preferable to "dry." But, if dry techniques are necessitated, cooking foods longer and at lower temperatures and marinated, basted or otherwise treated during cooking with citrus juices, vinegar and/or green herbs (e.g., rosemary, thyme, oregano, etc.) is preferable. **My recipes rely on cooking times, temperatures, and methods that help foods do as much for us as they can.** I also recognize that our real-world lives require us to do more than cook and eat. So my recipes not only incorporate healthy cooking techniques but also respect harried schedules. In part, The Young Skin Diet's recipes achieve this by ensuring that time in the kitchen is spent productively while slower-cooking foods steam, boil or poach. I also limit ingredient lists, while keeping the most powerful food combinations in play, and I keep cooking techniques simple and equipment needs basic.

As suggested earlier, for deeper knowledge of the relationships between particular foods' nutritional benefits and preparation techniques, I recommend perusing the recipes included in this book and reviewing the food lists provided.

Fifth, by making foods straightforward, delicious, and beautiful.

I think the best way to ensure we maintain good, healthy diets is by making those diets tasty and straightforward to prepare and eat. After all, sustainability is the key to diet success.

Recipes included in The Young Skin Diet have all been developed in the context of my own hectic and unpredictable life. I don't have the time or bandwidth to fuss over the minutiae that slow us down in the kitchen or bog us down at the table. And there's good reason for that: Nobody has the time or bandwidth to fuss in the kitchen. If I don't have tons of time, then neither do you. And The Young Skin Diet doesn't require it.

My recipes are straightforward. They're gratifying to make and satisfying to eat. They are attractive on the plate. They're balanced and nutritious even for those not specifically concerned with skin health. And, yes, they do your skin (and body) good along the way. My recommended foods can all be simply prepared and combined in pro-skin arrangements that taste great and are a joy to incorporate into your life. So even if my provided recipes are not specifically followed, they, along with the provided food lists, can give inspiration for implementing The Six Principles of The Young Skin Diet...deliciously.

After all, if we enjoy what we're cooking and eating, then our mouths and bodies can be happy – and that's a beautiful thing!

HOW TO USE THIS BOOK

The Young Skin Diet Calendar provides a suggested roadmap for when to make each of the prescribed recipes and treatments over a month-long period. The schedule is engineered to provide variety as well as balanced nutrition throughout each week and the month as a whole so that pro-skin nutrition is maximized over the course of the body's natural cycle of replenishing its skin cells. As a matter of practical benefit, the calendar also places preparation of simpler meals on weekdays. Though none of the recipes here are particularly difficult or time-consuming, those that are more involved are scheduled on weekends. And, recipes that yield multiple servings that can be preserved as leftovers are strategically placed to limit active preparatory work each day while still providing optimal skin-building nutrients throughout the program.

For days on which a particular meal slot does not have a specified recipe, "Build Your Own" recipes are available to plug in as desired. Build Your Own recipes need no more than 20 minutes of active prep and allow for flexibility to accommodate individual tastes and preferences as well as time constraints, budget considerations and caloric needs. As with all recipes included, Build Your Own recipes embody The Six Principles of The Young Skin Diet and accordingly call for ingredients and preparation techniques that are scientifically proven to be great for your skin. They just do so in a more "basic" way.

So, one way to adopt The Young Skin Diet is to simply follow the plan outlined in the provided calendar, recipes and Build Your Own charts. Since skin's regeneration cycle ranges from about one month to two months, it is important for best results to stick with the program at least through the provided calendar's scope and to subsequently maintain adherence to The Young Skin Diet's principles. After all, the longer you treat your skin right, the better it'll look and the longer it'll stay that way. That's the cumulative effect in action.

Inclusion of my recipes, the meal plans and treatment schedules is provided for general convenience and to facilitate following the program for best results:

- These elements are intended to make following a diet supportive of great skin easy and sustainable. The less we have to worry about what or how to do something, the more we can dedicate to actually doing it.
- They are meant to "jumpstart" your progress in adopting long-term habits that build healthy and youthful skin day by day.
- They are provided to illustrate The Six Principles of The Young Skin Diet,

demonstrating that these principles are real-world viable, can yield varied and fantastic tasting meals and, when used with regularity, result in healthier, younger-looking skin.

Incorporation of these recipes and plans is not meant to suggest, however, that these meals, treatments and combinations are the only way to employ The Six Principles of The Young Skin Diet. Rather, those six principles are elucidated so that you can find personalized ways to use them in your life for the long run. And the provided recipes can be used as illustrations of selections, combinations and preparations for tailored and adventurous eating. So long as the foods are compliant with the six principles, variety in diet is strongly beneficial for our health and skin!

It is in this regard that the recipes and skin treatments here can also be used "a la carte" if desired. Although results will be best if the program is adopted wholly, there are profound skin and health benefits to be enjoyed even if only a handful of these recipes and/or recommended foods replace traditional Western eating in your diet. In other words, you do not need to follow the outlined plan to a "t" in order to use The Young Skin Diet's principles to dramatically improve your skin.

Remember: This is a "no-fail" diet plan. You can achieve younger skin as long as The Six Priniciples of The Young Skin Diet are generally adopted – the more they are adhered to, the tastier and greater the results will be. It's that simple. So, you can use the recommended food lists and everyday practice as the foundation of a successful implementation of The Young Skin Diet even if none of the provided recipes is used. Even still, I'd recommend checking out each recipe for ideas on good-for-you skin ingredients, combinations and preparations and science findings underpinning them. See the next page for a couple of illustrations outlining the various components of each recipe in The Young Skin Diet.

NO-MORE-DARK-SPOTS OATS

½ cup gluten-free rolled oats, dry	Place dry oats in a small bowl. Do not cook.
1 tsp. unrefined coconut oil, melted	Stir in coconut oil, honey, cinnamon, and chia seeds. Top with blueberries, pomegranate seeds, and walnuts. Serve.
2 tsp. honey	
¼ tsp. cinnamon	
½ tsp. chia seeds	
¼ cup blueberries	
2 tbsp. pomegranate seeds	
5 to 10 walnuts, roughly chopped	

SCIENCE & NUTRITION

Blueberries: Blueberries are a natural source of arbutin, a powerful skin lightener that is effective at reducing pigmentation inconsistencies in skin. Arbutin is similar in structure (and convertible to) hydroquinone, the active ingredient in popular skin-lightening creams.

- Seo, D., et al. "Biotechnological production of arbutins (a- and β-arbutins), skin lightening agents, and their derivatives," Applied Microbiology and Biotechnology. 2012 Sep.; 95(6): 1417-1425.
- Jeon, J., et al. "Simultaneous determination of arbutin and its decomposed product hydroquinone in whitening creams using high-performance liquid chromatography with photodiode array detection: effect of temperature and pH on decomposition," International Journal of Cosmetic Science. 2015.

Pomegranate Seeds: The ellagic acid found in pomegranate seeds has been found effective at reducing and treating UV-induced photodamage, thus helping resolve a main factor in skin aging and the production of dark spots in skin.

- Hseu, Y., et al. "Ellagic acid protects human keratinocyte (HaCaT) cells against UVA-induced oxidative stress and apoptosis through the upregulation of the HO-1 and Nrf-2 antioxidant genes," Food and Chemical Toxicology. 2012 May; 50(5): 1245-1255.

460 calories; 26g fat; 7g sat. fat; 0mg cholesterol; 10mg sodium; 210mg potassium; 52g carbohydrates; 9g fiber; 19g sugar; 11g protein. 1 serving.

> **All ingredients are selected for pro-skin benefits.**

> Preparation techniques are specifically designed to enhance – not degrade – foods' benefits for healthy, young skin.

> **Science describes some of the research basis for what makes the recipe great for young skin.**

> Citations are provided for follow on reading if desired.

> **Especially potent pro-skin combinations are often called out in the science section of a recipe.**

YOUNG SKIN CURRY SOUP

2 tsp. unrefined coconut oil	Heat coconut oil in a large stockpot over medium to medium-high heat. Add onion and sauté until translucent, about 2 minutes. Add remaining vegetables, ginger and spices. Sauté for 2 more minutes.
½ cup red onion, chopped	
2 cups carrots, peeled and sliced into ¼-inch rounds	Add vegetable stock and bring to a boil. Reduce heat to simmer, cover and cook until vegetables are tender, about 35 to 45 minutes. Stir in coconut milk.
2 cups sweet potatoes, cut into ½-inch cubes with skin left on	Transfer pot contents in 2 to 3 batches to a food processor. Pulse until smooth. Serve immediately.
½ tbsp. ginger, peeled and grated	
1 tsp. cumin	
½ tsp. coriander	
½ tsp. allspice	
¼ tsp. salt	
¼ tsp. cinnamon	
3 cups low-sodium vegetable broth	
1 cup low fat coconut milk	

SCIENCE & NUTRITION

Red Onion: With stronger free radical scavenging activity than yellow onion or even garlic, red onion provides significant antioxidant action in the body to promote healthy, youthful skin.

- Nuutila, A.M., et al. "Comparison of antioxidant activities of onion and garlic extracts by inhibition of lipid peroxidation and radical scavenging activity," Food Chemistry. 2003 Jun.; 81(4): 485-493.
- Prakash, D. "Antioxidant and free radical scavenging activities of phenols from onion (allium cepa)," Food Chemistry. 2007; 102(4): 1389-1393.

Ginger + Cumin + Coriander + Allspice + Cinnamon: Spices, including those used here, provide concentrated and varied antioxidants, which remove the precursors of oxidative damage and skin aging from the body. Antioxidant activity of these spices is enhanced by cooking them in a soup preparation involving long heating times.

- Yanishlieva, N., et al. "Natural antioxidants from herbs and spices," European Journal of Lipid Science and Technology. 2006 Sep.; 108(9): 776-793.
- Khatum, M., et al. "Effect of thermal treatment on radical-scavenging activity of some spices," Food Science and Technology Research. 2006; 12(3): 178-185.

As someone who has a family and worked in high-stakes consulting for over a decade, I know how pressed for time schedules can become, particularly once overtime, commutes and caring for other family members are incorporated into the work week. I also know that careers regularly invade weekend time.

Happily, this doesn't mean there isn't room for eating a diet that builds great, youthful skin. Over the years, I've developed easy ways to make healthy eating a sustainable, simple habit. Here are some tips to help you follow The Young Skin Diet and make young-skin eating a permanent part of your existence.

Plan Ahead

Plan your meals for the week. Every week. For me, this is the most important element in maintaining a healthy eating regimen. I'm most likely to stray from healthy eating when I don't have a plan, particularly when I'm ravenous at the end of a long day and have to try making a good decision about what to eat. Am I the only one who finds thinking clearly on an empty stomach to be borderline impossible? Planning ahead takes game-time thinking out of the equation.

That's not to say I don't enjoy an occasional "cheat meal." I incorporate an indulgence or two into my weekly meal planning. For example, I'll enjoy an occasional night out at, say, a steakhouse with my family or have a glass of wine. This practice keeps things fresh and, more often than not, serves as a powerful reminder of how good I feel when I do eat according to my six principles.

In my opinion, the occasional indulgence is critical to long-term, sustained success with a diet. The operative word there is *occasional*. If you do happen to overindulge, don't beat yourself up. Acknowledge and accept it, get back on track, and move on. The next time the urge to stray sneaks up on you, try to envision a conversation with your future self in which you explain the transgression – one that your "current" self enjoys and your "future" self pays the price for. That sort of exercise is a very powerful behavioral economics trick – give it a try.

When planning meals for the week, I always take into account upcoming commitments. If my mornings are going to be rushed during a particular week, I'll plan to make my Build Your Own Breakfast oatmeal recipes for breakfast. If my evenings will be packed with summer activities, I make sure I have leftovers on hand or the ingredients for one of the quick-hit Build Your Own Combo recipes for more filling fare. All my Build Your Own Combo recipes can be made with 20 minutes or less active prep – just like most of my other recipes – so they take even less time than dashing to the nearest fast food restaurant for takeout.

One final note on planning: plan what sounds good to you and your family. If you're not excited about what you're eating, you won't stick with it. **The Build Your Own charts are included in The Young Skin Diet to give you the flexibility and freedom to choose easy meals that sound good while still keeping your diet on track!** They also take some of the work out of planning meals for the week, so use them.

Make Weekly Grocery Shopping a Habit

With all that meal planning, you'll have to visit the grocery store, something I enjoy doing but I know others view as a chore. Here are my tips for making grocery shopping a little less painful.

If you finish work early on Friday, stay at the office for 5 extra minutes to write a grocery list and swing by the store on the way home. Stores are usually quiet and fully stocked on Friday afternoon, and it'll cause minimal disruption to your weekend. Alternatively, go first thing Saturday morning since stores are similarly quiet and fully stocked first thing on Saturday. Plus, it will help you get your shopping out of the way so that it's not looming over your head all weekend.

Whatever you do, **don't wait until the Sunday evening rush!** Your shopping will take twice as long and items will be picked over. And if you're not used to doing a weekly grocery run, you may burn out before giving it a fair shot.

When possible, divide and conquer. During my family's weekly trip the store, my role is to select produce. My husband picks up packaged products like eggs, orange juice, canned fish and the like. This sort of division of labor works to our relative competencies. Cartons and cans can be heavy to pick up and lug around, so it's a great job for my husband. And I'm patient enough to sort through bunches of produce to select the really good ones.

If your kids are old enough roam the aisles alone, give them some items to pick up as well. Shopping goes by much faster if you can divide and conquer, and kids (like spouses) love to feel helpful. An easy way to organize things is to e-mail the shopping list to each member of your family before heading out the door. I write each person's name on the list and what they're supposed to pick up under their name. You can even add a little fun by seeing who can pick up their items the fastest. The winner gets bragging rights all week long.

Once they get the hang of things, try writing your shopping list by aisle, so that everybody's not running across the store – though that can be exciting!

Not convinced you want to commit to meal planning and shopping? Think about the savings. The dollar cost of every meal made at home is a fraction of the price of eating the same meal out, and the savings of eating just one additional meal at home per week instead of going out can add up quickly. For a family of four, the weekly savings can be as high as $35 per meal. That's **over $1,800 per year saved by choosing to replace one meal per week out with a home-cooked one!** Who knew looking good could be so enriching?

Have "Go-Tos"

I like to think of my go-tos as my no-brainer options. They are healthy, easy-to-no-prep options for every meal that I enjoy eating. Plus, they make the task of writing a grocery list fly by. Go-tos quickly take up spots in the week and remove a good deal of pressure from meal planning.

So what are some good examples of go-to foods? Gluten-free rolled oats, orange juice, tea, and eggs are often my go-to breakfast ingredient options since they're healthy and can easily be arranged a number of ways. See my Build Your Own Breakfast chart for quick, easy, delicious morning recipes.

Both my Build Your Own Breakfast and Build Your Own Combo charts contain recipes that are easy to make from basic ingredients: they all make perfect go-tos. Though some of these dishes may rely upon similar ingredients, different spices and preparation techniques cause the flavors to be unique while retaining young-skin benefits. Because you won't always feel like eating the same type of dish, I've designed tasty, palate-pleasing Build Your Own dishes that comply with The Six Principles of The Young Skin Diet.

At lunchtime, salads that are easy to pack and take to the office, like those in my Build Your Own Combo chart, are favorites. Also great are make-ahead options that can be used for several days like my Young Skin Curry Soup.

For sides or snacks, I like to have my Revitalizing Goji Greatness on hand. I also love easy-to-transport, no-fuss fruits like apples, which can be quickly transformed to my great-tasting Collagen-Building Pomme Snack. Combinations of fruits and nuts are particularly powerful as agents of young skin, so I make a point of picking them up whenever my home supplies run low for quick and easy snacking compliant with The Six Principles of The Young Skin Diet.

When I need dinner in a dash, I often look to the recipes on the heartier side of my Build Your Own Combo chart, where everything is extremely simple to plan and make and tastes delicious.

Reconsider Leftovers

Seriously. Leftovers are often my savior, and I can't understand why they're not prized by everyone for the economical and easy option they are. Weeks get busy and I get tired, so it's often the case that I don't feel like making dinner. Having leftovers that I can reheat is wonderful. I know I have a healthy, tasty, affordable option that keeps my eating on track and my budget in check.

The Young Skin Diet calendar incorporates leftovers into your week to keep meal prep to a minimum and to accommodate busy schedules

Can't stomach the thought of eating leftovers? Try "repurposing" your food. For example, it's easy to make delicious lettuce-wrapped fish tacos out of my Anti-Wrinkle Spiced Salmon leftovers or crudités dip from leftover salad dressing from my Elasticity Boost Asian Fusion Salad.

Alternatively, some foods may be frozen and saved for enjoyment on a later date. My Young Skin Curry Soup, The Ageless Ms. Fit Burger, and the Build Your Own Breakfast quinoa and oat bran recipes, among others, can be frozen and saved for a hectic day that calls for a quick meal that adheres to the six principles.

Rotate Favorites

One key to healthy eating is variety, not only in the foods you eat but the way in which they are prepared. You can make meal planning, shopping, and prep a bit easier while still maintaining variety if you have some favorite meals that your family regularly rotates through.

As an example, a favorite, easy meal in my household is my Stress-Fighting Salmon Cakes. However, as much as we love eating them, I try to make sure we don't have them more than once every other week, or even as infrequently as once a month. This keeps the recipe fresh and exciting, and keeps variety high.

The month-long calendar in The Young Skin Diet was designed with this in mind. Even if the month-long calendar were followed exactly month-in and month-out for a year, each recipe would only be prepared 12 times, leaving plenty of room for variety and no such thing as "the usual."

Use The Young Skin Diet "Strategies for Success" to make adoption of the plan even simpler. Plan ahead, make weekly grocery shopping a habit, have "go-tos," reconsider leftovers and rotate favorites.

With The Young Skin Diet's calendar, recipes, "Build Your Own" charts, and strategies for success, you're well on your way to eating a healthy diet that builds young skin.

The following additional resources will be helpful in condensing The Young Skin Diet's recommendations into broad guidance regarding ingredient selection. Included is a list of general food categories and brief description of which foods within each category are, and are not, recommended as part of The Young Skin Diet. Following each description is a listing of exemplar foods used in various recipes included in this book that promote great, young-looking skin. Additionally, a high-level list of everyday practices that can be helpful in incorporating the Six Principles of The Young Skin Diet into your life is set forth.

Fruits

All fruits are recommended. A total of 6 to 8 fruit and vegetable servings should be consumed per day.

Emphasis should be placed on organically grown and unprocessed selections. A wide variety and different combinations of fruits are best.

Frozen fruits can be excellent alternatives to fresh fruits since they can enable greater variety and organic choices, particularly during calendar periods outside of harvest times. In addition, they maintain their nutritional profile at least as well as fresh varieties.

The majority of fruits, with the notable exception of tomatoes, are most nutritious when uncooked. Among fruits that must be processed prior to human consumption, especially olives, **look for minimal processing**, as in kalamata olives. For tomato products, also find those with minimal processing and minimal added ingredients.

Note that fruit juices, even juices made at home, are less beneficial than whole fruits (and may even be detrimental) since fibers can be lost during the juicing process, while sugars are retained. Store-bought juices also often have added sugars and preservatives that can be detrimental. **Should fruit juices be desired, citrus juices, especially varieties containing pulp and no added sugars, may be best.**

Exemplar fruits in the provided recipes with interesting young skin benefits include:

- **Strawberries:** chemicals found in strawberries inhibit the formation of advanced glycation end products, which degrade the body's tissues, including skin collagen.
- **Cherries:** anthocyanins, serotonin and melatonin from cherries all provide pro-skin health benefits, including anti-inflammation and pro-sleep effects.
- **Goji berries:** the release of so-called progenitor cells, believed to have a key role in maintaining the vitality of the body's systems, including skin, is promoted by goji berries.
- **Red grapes:** resveratrol, found only in red grapes, is a powerful anti-aging antioxidant.
- **Blueberries:** arbutin found in blueberries is a powerful skin lightener that can help resolve dark spots.

Combinations of fruits, and combinations of fruits with vegetables, nuts, eggs and poultry, are strongly recommended. Herbs and spices also can enhance the pro-skin benefits of fruits and are accordingly advised to be added to fruits.

Vegetables

Most vegetables are recommended. (See "Starches and Grains" and "Legumes" sections below for discussion related to vegetables that are not recommended.)

Emphasis should be placed on organically grown and unprocessed selections. A wide variety and different combinations of vegetables are best.

Frozen vegetables can be excellent alternatives to fresh vegetables since they can enable greater variety and organic choices, particularly during calendar periods outside of harvest times. In addition, they maintain their nutritional profile at least as well as fresh varieties.

Some vegetables' nutritional values are enhanced by cooking, while others are diminished. As a very broad guideline (to which there are exceptions), green and leafy vegetables (e.g., kale, broccoli, etc.) are most nutritious when consumed raw or when cooking times are limited. Colorful vegetables (e.g., carrots, bell peppers, etc.) often exhibit nutritional gains during cooking.

Vegetable juices, even juices made at home, are less beneficial than whole vegetables (and may even be detrimental). Store-bought juices also often have added salts, sugars and preservatives that can be detrimental. **Should juices** with vegetable-like flavor characteristics be desired, low sodium tomato juice may be best because of tomatoes' particularly good responses to processing.

Exemplar vegetables in the provided recipes with interesting young skin benefits include:

- **Cabbage:** the isoflavonoid equol found in cabbage is a potent antioxidant that helps promote collagen and elastin levels and wound healing.
- **Cucumber:** bioaccessible silica in cucumber is used directly in collagen formation.
- **Asparagus:** the vegetable's protection against skin wrinkling has been clinically demonstrated.
- **Beets:** particularly damaging hydroxyl radicals are scavenged by beets' antioxidants.
- **Garlic:** the allicin antioxidant in garlic is especially strong, and garlic has been shown to inhibit advanced glycation end product formation.

Combinations of vegetables, and combinations of vegetables with fruits, nuts, eggs and poultry, are strongly recommended. Herbs and spices also can enhance the pro-skin benefits of vegetables and are accordingly advised to be added to vegetables.

Starches and Grains

Some starchy vegetables and some grains are recommended, while others are not.

Sweet potatoes, peas and squash are recommended because of their beneficial nutrient profiles for skin.

White potatoes and corn, on the other hand, are not recommended.

Quinoa, gluten-free rolled oats and wild rice are the best grains for accordance with The Six Principles of The Young Skin Diet and the science of skin health. However, because one of the guiding philosophies of The Young Skin Diet is that diet sustainability is enabled by great taste and because certain foods with especially strong pro-skin benefits taste best with white rice, a couple of my recipes include white rice. (Note that, in the debate between whether white rice or brown rice is superior, there is no clear winner. Since the flavors of white rice are preferable in the dishes in which it is called for, I include it rather than brown rice in recipes where rice is needed and where wild rice will not suffice.) On its own, white rice is not recommended.

Gluten-containing grains, including wheat, barley and rye, are not recommended since, as with corn and white potatoes, any nutritional and culinary values from these foods can be either equally or better provided by other foods without the former foods' allergenic downsides.

Starches and grains in the provided recipes with interesting young skin benefits include:

- **Sweet potato:** the abundant vitamin A in sweet potatoes is used by the skin to protect collagen from degradation and to rebuild collagen.
- **Quinoa:** lysine is an amino acid often missing from plant sources but found in quinoa; accordingly, quinoa presents a complete protein, as well as beneficial vitamins like vitamin E, all of which benefits skin youth.
- **Gluten-free rolled oats:** beta-glucans found in oats help control growth and metabolic action in the skin and help fight skin infections.

Recommended starches and grains can best be exploited for their pro-skin benefits when combined with other recommended food categories like fruits and vegetables, oils, eggs, fish and shellfish. As with other food categories, the use of spices and herbs to complement recommended starches and grains is advised.

Legumes

Some legumes are recommended and some are not. In general, since some individuals exhibit digestive difficulty with legumes that would be expected to render adherence to the diet unsustainable, **my recommendation of any legumes as part of The Young Skin Diet stems from those specified foods' particularly beneficial nutritional profiles vis-à-vis young skin.**

Green beans, peas (as discussed above), chickpeas (i.e., garbanzo beans) and black beans are recommended for their strong pro-skin health nutritional profiles. Other types of beans provide lower levels of pro-skin benefits like hyaluronic acid and anthocyanin antioxidants and are thus not recommended.

Lentils, which are used in cuisine in ways similar to some beans, starchy vegetables and grains, are not recommended since their nutritional profile is less advantageous than some foods like chickpeas that can function similarly in dishes.

Peanuts, which can cause allergenic responses in some individuals and the nutritional benefits of which can be readily provided by other foods with lower allergy rates, are not recommended.

Legumes in the provided recipes with interesting young skin benefits include:

- **Green beans:** abundant in highly bioavailable silica, green beans directly support collagen.
- **Chickpeas:** hyaluronic acid found in chickpeas keeps the collagen matrix of the skin healthy and volumized.

As with other recommended food categories, combining legumes with other foods is advisable for maximizing the foods' young-skin benefits.

Nuts and Seeds

A variety of nuts and seeds is recommended for their good fats, vitamins and minerals. Each day, at least 1 serving, but no more than 3 servings, of nuts and seeds should be consumed.

Exemplar nuts and seeds in the provided recipes with interesting young skin benefits include:

- **Chia seeds:** ALA Omega-3 fatty acids found in chia seeds are anti-inflammatory and promote cellular function in the skin.
- **Pistachios:** the phenolic compounds in pistachios fight inflammation and free radicals, while pistachios' fats support various metabolic functions in the skin.
- **Pumpkin seeds:** varied tocopherols, including vitamin E, are abundant in pumpkin seeds and are believed to behave synergistically with one another in eradicating oxidative stress.
- **Pomegranate seeds:** ellagic acid in pomegranate seeds reduces and resolves UV photodamage.

Particularly in combination with fruits, grains and starches, and spices and herbs, the skin-enhancing credentials of nuts and seeds can most readily be exploited.

Oils

Extra virgin olive oil and unrefined coconut oil are recommended. Extra virgin olive oil has some of the highest levels of good skin and pro-health benefits among oils, while unrefined coconut oil retains its healthy constituents that are vastly reduced by the process used to make refined coconut oil.

Vegetable oils are not recommended.

Extra virgin olive oil and unrefined coconut oil have demonstrated proskin health benefits, while other oils like vegetable oils do not (or have been shown to harm skin).

Oils included in the provided recipes are:

- **Olive oil:** reductions In the rate and severity of skin photoaging, and increases in skin elasticity, are linked with the consumption of olive oil.
- **Coconut oil:** the lauric acid in coconut oil fights infection that can manifest in skin and damage tissues.

Cooking with these recommended oils is advisable for enhancing other foods' pro-skin benefits, including all other recommended food categories.

Spices and Herbs

All spices and herbs, excluding salt, are recommended. They should be used, with variety, often.

Spices and herbs provide concentrated antioxidant and other benefits for healthy skin, and their overall nutrition and flavor profiles make them excellent for enhancing other foods' nutrition and taste. Spices and herbs along with vinegars and citrus juices also help protect foods during cooking. Notwithstanding their benefits, individual spices and herbs should be used in moderation since, at high levels, some may have deleterious health consequences.

Because of the way I use it in my cooking and provided recipes, I include honey in this category of foods. Honey, in moderation, is recommended for its nutritional value to skin and its variety of culinary applications. Other added sugars should be limited as much as possible and are not recommended.

It should be noted here that, in a couple of my provided recipes, I call for small amounts of palm sugar as means of achieving the right flavor balance in the dish. However, my recipes, including these, counteract any added sugars from honey or palm sugar with high fiber values. Consider the following: **In the U.S., the average total sugar to total fiber ratio in the diet is about 12, and the ratio of *added* sugars alone to total fiber is over 7. My recipes collectively have a total sugar to total fiber ratio of less than 3 (considered by some commentators to be approximately optimal), providing a substantially improved ratio from typical levels while still providing excellent flavor.** What this ratio means is that, for every 3 grams of sugar included collectively in recipes provided in The Young Skin Diet, there is at least 1 gram of fiber also included.

In this same vein, some researchers recommend diets in which the ratio of total carbohydrates to total fiber in the diet is 10 or lower. (This line of research

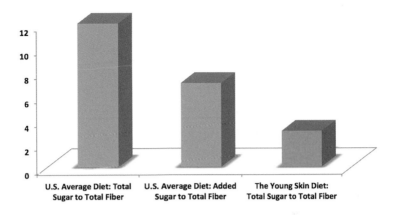

Sugar-Fiber Ratio:
U.S. Average and The Young Skin Diet

has been specifically linked with "whole grain" food selection.) **Recipes in The Young Skin Diet collectively yield a total carbohydrate to total fiber ratio of less than 7.** That is, for every 7 grams of total carbohydrates provided in recipes in this book, those recipes also collectively provide at least 1 gram of fiber. In the average diet in the U.S., there are about *12 grams of sugar alone* consumed per 1 gram of fiber in the diet (and total carbohydrates per gram of fiber are even higher).

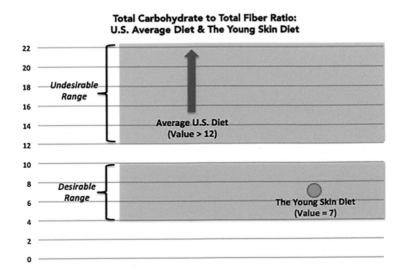

Total Carbohydrate to Total Fiber Ratio:
U.S. Average Diet & The Young Skin Diet

Regarding salt, it is not recommended to add salt to foods. However, in a limited number of recipes provided in this book, I call for small amounts of salt in the ingredients list as means of balancing overall flavor. My recipes also emphasize potassium to offset any detrimental effects of these minimal salt additions. **While the average American diet exhibits a potassium to sodium ratio of about 0.7, researchers have identified an optimal ratio of between 3 and 4. The Young Skin Diet's recipes collectively provide a ratio of just over 3.1.**

Exemplar spices and herbs in the provided recipes with interesting young skin benefits include:

- **Rosemary:** like other herbs, rosemary helps protect fats from oxidation and inhibits the formation of advanced glycation end products.
- **Mint:** oils found in mint have potent anti-inflammatory, antiviral and antibacterial properties that help keep skin healthy.
- **Allspice:** the antioxidant activity of allspice has been shown to support processes including collagen production in the skin.
- **Turmeric:** curcumin compounds in turmeric are powerful anti-inflammatory agents.

Dairy

Dairy is not recommended because of its potential as an allergen and because any nutritional value from dairy can be easily obtained elsewhere in a varied diet.

Coconut milk is a preferred substitute for milk.

Coconut milk, as part of The Young Skin Diet, behaves similarly to coconut oil and is recommended for use in similar applications, particularly as a part of multi-component recipes that benefit from coconut's fatty acid profile.

PREBIOTICS & PROBIOTICS

There is lots of marketing these days of products offering probiotic benefits. Why don't probiotics feature more prominently in The Young Skin Diet? Summarily because the science is unsettled on probiotics. For example, probiotic foods like yogurt introduce bacteria to the gut; however, the composition and population of every person's gut bacteria is unique, and probiotics may not be ideal in one-size-fits-all types of introductions – there's little research indicating the effects of introducing bacteria to the gut in diversity or composition dissimilar from the initial population. Prebiotics, on the other hand, use fiber-rich foods to feed a person's existing gut bacteria, enabling support of the gut microbiome in a way that fits everyone individually – and fiber-rich foods are a very big part of The Young Skin Diet. Garlic, onion, asparagus, and bananas are just a few examples of foods that contain prebiotics and which are included in the provided recipes.

Meat

Red meats and pork are not recommended because of their myriad skin-harming effects.

In small amounts, poultry is recommended because of the importance of carnosine and complete proteins in a diet supportive of young skin.

Recall that poultry consumption implies the introduction of more AGEs to the diet. Consuming poultry is accordingly recommended when AGE-fighting preparation and cooking techniques are used (i.e., "wet" cooking techniques and the strategic use of AGE-reducing herbs, spices and marinades).

Eggs

Eggs are recommended for their protein, antioxidants, beneficial fats and positive interactions with other foods.

Eggs from hens fed diets supportive of EPA and DHA Omega-3 fatty acids are specifically recommended.

Eggs can be particularly beneficial for young skin when combined with fruits, vegetables and herbs and spices.

Fish and Shellfish

Some fish and shellfish are recommended, while some are not.

Wild-caught salmon, sardines, anchovies, barramundi and wild-caught shrimp are recommended for their beneficial fatty acid profiles, protein, anti-inflammation effects and antioxidant profiles.

Other types of fish are not recommended because they:
1. do not provide significant or beneficial ratios of Omega-3 fats;
2. contain harmful mercury levels (e.g., tuna, some mackerel, etc.);
3. contain harmful antibiotics or other pollutants (e.g., farmed salmon); or

4. have other significant downsides that outweigh any benefits.

Exemplar fish and shellfish in the provided recipes with interesting young skin benefits include:

- **Wild-caught salmon:** EPA and DHA long-chain Omega-3 fatty acids are particularly plentiful in salmon and benefit the body's entire ecosystem with inflammation-fighting action that helps preserve skin health.
- **Wild shrimp:** astaxanthin and selenium in shrimp improve skin tone and texture and enhance resistance to UV photoaging.

Strategic combination with vegetables, herbs and spices and grains and starches can maximize the pro-skin benefits of recommended fish and shellfish.

Beverages

Sufficient water intake is crucial. A daily intake of 64 ounces is a good starting point for ensuring sufficient water intake.

Teas of all kinds are recommended for their skin-related benefits. Teas should be home-brewed, not purchased bottled or canned.

Coffee is not recommended because of tea's easy substitutability for coffee and tea's stronger benefits for skin.

Alcoholic beverages are not recommended (despite beers' highly bio-available silica levels), nor are carbonated drinks or, as previously described, most fruit or vegetable juices.

EVERYDAY PRACTICES FOR YOUNG SKIN

This list of everyday practices is meant to help you incorporate The Six Principles of The Young Skin Diet into your life, regardless of whether you choose to follow the provided meal plans and recipes or you choose to build younger skin by modifying your existing dietary routines in other ways. Though not comprehensive, this list of everyday practices will help keep you on the path to healthy, young skin.

1. **Upon waking each morning, drink at least 8 ounces of cold water.** This practice gets your daily hydration goals off to a good start and addresses overnight moisture loss. Moreover, the water helps power your body's overall metabolic activity and helps cleanse waste from cells, which collectively helps keep skin clear and supple.

2. **Drink tea each morning.** Adding to your hydration levels and providing a potent allowance of antioxidants and anti-inflammatories, tea ensures your great-skin day gets off to a fast start. Remember to add a squeeze of lemon to amplify tea's healthy skin benefits.

3. **Eat at least 6 to 8 servings of fruits and vegetables each day.** This is crucial for great skin since plant-based foods are the strongest single-source bearers of antioxidants, anti-inflammatories, hydrating moisture, minerals and vitamins in the diet. The easiest way to meet this goal, which is based upon the serving threshold at which skin benefits are most likely to be quickly realized, is to consume fruits and vegetables as follows:
   - Eat at least one serving during each day's 3 principal meals (i.e., breakfast, lunch and dinner). This practice, which is very easy to do, provides at least 3 daily servings toward your goal.
   - Eat at least one serving during each day's 3 snack times (i.e., mid-morning, afternoon and bedtime). This practice adds at least 3 more daily servings.
   - Once per day, consume either lunch or dinner that is vegan or vegetarian. This practice increases the likelihood that at least 2 servings of fruits and/or vegetables are consumed during the

meal. Following this practice sums with the others to provide more than 6 daily servings of fruits and vegetables.

- When eating fruits and vegetables, recall the research findings presented elsewhere in this book to reap the maximum additive and synergistic pro-skin rewards from each serving. Consuming fruits together with nuts or seeds, and with spices is beneficial, while consuming raw vegetables with eggs and using appropriate preparation techniques ensures maximum skin benefits.

4. **Eat at least 1 serving (but not more than 3 servings) of nuts and/ or seeds per day.** The easiest and most beneficially pro-skin practice to meet this goal is to sprinkle a serving of nuts or seeds atop fruit for a snack. As outlined in the research discussed elsewhere in this book, nuts and seeds often exhibit strong additive and synergistic pro-skin benefits when consumed alongside fruit. At least one daily serving ensures receipt of nuts'/seeds' young skin benefits, while limiting the daily intake to 3 or fewer ensures their relatively high caloric and fat content will not cause overall dietary imbalance.

5. **Eat a serving of recommended fish at least 2 times per week, and more frequently if possible.** The pro-health and skin building credentials of properly selected and prepared fish are excellent, most notably those connected with greater Omega-3 fats balance in the diet – an effect most directly achieved with fish consumption (and reduction in processed food consumption). And, since most meats are not recommended (save an occasional serving of properly selected and prepared poultry), fish can provide the tactile and flavor satisfaction of meats while providing excellent young skin benefits. Recall that "wet" cooking of fish is best.

6. **As much as possible, consume organic and/or wild, rather than conventionally farmed, produce, grains and other foods.** The pesticide, herbicide and other chemicals found in conventionally farmed foods can cause a host of issues that erode skin quality and deplete foods of some of their pro-health benefits.

7. **Avoid all processed foods, red meats, pork, wheat, gluten, dairy (including products containing lactose or casein), soy, corn, peanuts and added salts or sugars.** By avoiding processed foods, which often contain dozens of ingredients (not to mention imbalanced fats), this practice is simple. When habits urge you to eat an unhealthy snack, opt instead for fruits, vegetables, nuts and/or seeds. These pro-skin alternatives satisfy the salty/sweet/crunchy/quick needs that cause us to crave processed foods that harm and age our skin. As a bonus, these alternatives are fantastic for building young skin.

8. **As much as possible, use "wet" cooking techniques and limit cooking times of vegetables, particularly green and leafy vegetables.** This practice also applies to most fruits; though, from a practical perspective, cooking time and temperature are less of a concern for fruits, with the notable exception of tomatoes, which can benefit from cooking. For fish, eggs and poultry (and any other animal-based food, for that matter), cook using "wet" cooking methods and low heat. High-heat grilling, baking, roasting and the like of animal products should be avoided. This practice limits AGE formation and enables foods to retain more of their pro-skin nutritional elements.

9. **Limit your cooking oils to just extra virgin olive oil and unrefined virgin coconut oil.** These oils exhibit pro-skin benefits, while most other cooking oils can harm skin.

10. **Use spices, excluding sugars and salt, regularly in meals and snacks.** Spices add flavor and allow you to realize pro-skin health benefits from their antioxidants and anti-inflammatories.

11. **Eat regularly throughout the day.** This helps keep your body's nutritional needs satisfied, allows pro-skin building blocks to always be on hand for optimal skin health, and helps reduce the likelihood of hunger urges that cause you to stray from pro-skin eating. Even if not following the particular recipes and meal plans set out in this book, the provided calendars show an eating schedule reflecting one meal or snack approximately every 3 hours that can be readily followed.

12. **Permit yourself to treat your skin with external moisturizers, ex-foliants, antioxidants and anti-inflammatories free from chemicals and preservatives (as with my provided skin treatment "recipes") once per day.** And always wear sunscreen, preferably mineral-based lotions using zinc oxide.

SURPRISES FROM MY RESEARCH

My analysis of food, nutrition and skin was eye opening and, in many ways quite surprising. My surprise at the six themes I uncovered stemmed from three observations.

First, the general themes I found are quite simple – we can eat for great skin without excessively complex formulas or schemes. Despite what some of the popular diet trends would lead us to believe, the overwhelming scientific evidence is that the prescription for great eating is pretty straightforward. There are certain foods best if avoided, and certain best practices, which I've outlined; but we don't need to make exaggerated departures from socially acceptable behavior to nourish our skin and bodies properly.

Second, the foods that are best for our skin and the foods that are best for our overall health substantially overlap. When you consider how integrated they body's various systems, including skin, are, that fact is admittedly not so surprising. But it is a powerful observation and so bears repeating: Even if there are some foods that might service our skins' needs more efficiently than others (and those foods are certainly part of The Young Skin Diet), it can generally be stated that, if we eat foods that are great for our skin, we're also eating foods excellent for general health, and vice versa.

This observation implies a pair of corollaries. For one, we can rest assured that The Young Skin Diet does not outline an eating plan that nourishes our skin at the expense of our overall heath. Additionally, we can reasonably expect any dish in The Young Skin Diet plan to be a great part of anyone's diet, even if they're not specifically interested in improving the vitality of their skin's appearance.

The recommended foods, combination and preparation techniques, meal plans, recipes and treatments outlined in The Young Skin Diet are specifically engineered to most directly and efficaciously enhance your skin's appearance and youthfulness. Every selection and combination is tailor-made to the task of improving skin as rapidly and fully as possible. And they also benefit overall health, particularly relative to most Western eating habits.

The third thing that surprised me about what my research uncovered is that more people in Western society don't already eat a diet more conducive to great skin and overall health.

There's simply no good reason not to eat foods that ensure our skin stays youthful and our bodies stay lean. The foods that provide these benefits are better tasting, more attractive, more satisfying and often less expensive than the unhealthy – even lethal – foods that comprise most Westerners' daily diets. So what gives?

Even if there's no good reason we don't eat what we should, that doesn't mean there's no reason at all. Our society is more exhausted, more likely to be obese, more inclined to have diabetes, less likely to be satisfied with life and less physically capable because, according to demographic, expenditure and calorie consumption data I've reviewed, it appears we've become addicted to two things.

Our first addiction is the quick-hit simple carbohydrates that are infused in many, many processed foods. According to the USDA Economic Research Service, as of 2009, 63% of the calories consumed by Americans came from processed foods, encompassing added fats, sugars and refined grains. Roughly two-thirds! Although the study is a few years old, data suggest the proportion of these "bad" calories is on the rise over time, so it's not likely the current numbers are any better.

Calories in the U.S. Average Diet: Highly Processed

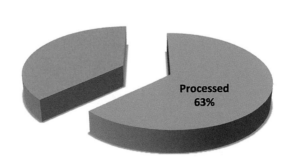

Processed
63%

One reason we seem to be addicted to these bad calories is that they stimulate the pleasure centers in our brains. These processed ingredients set off a cascade of biological events that harm our long-term health but give us fast, though fleeting, pleasure. We repeatedly undermine our long-run health and the youthfulness of our skin to receive momentary gratification from added processed fats, excess sugars and refined grain carbohydrates (none of which is part of The Young Skin Diet!).

It's drug addiction, plain and simple. The problem is that it's so easy to get our hands on these drugs, it can be very difficult to not take a "hit." And, after a long period of repeated exposure to them, we can actually feel ill without them in our system…even as our system punishes our skin and bodies for the abuse.

What's worse is that, as we become accustomed to the feel-good hits, we seek out more and more offending foods in increasingly rapid frequency. When we "OD" on processed foods and simple carbohydrates, we become diabetic, overweight, sluggish, clouded and temperamental, and we lose the natural glow that makes us look our best. Indeed, simple carbohydrates like added fructose are a main culprit in promoting oxidative stress and inflammation in the body that precipitate aged-looking skin.

Our second addiction is to "no-effort convenience." According to a paper written by economists in the USDA Economic Research Service, around 90 percent of us living in the U.S. make purchases of convenience foods (representing a dramatic increase over time), with most of us indicating our convenience food purchases occur because we're "too worn out to cook in the evenings." This addiction is perhaps even more insidious than that of processed ingredients since the relationship between our yearning for no-effort ease and the foods we eat is more complex.

Yes, we all lead busy lives. And yes, convenience foods such as fast food, microwave dinners and the like can save the day in a pinch. I've been there!

But more often than not, our reliance on no-effort convenience foods stems from the fact that we get "too worn out" during the day *too easily*. By dinnertime, the last thing we want to think about is making a meal when we can just pop that premade burrito in the microwave and call it good. The reason we don't want to think about making dinner, and the reason we get worn out so easily, is because we're often systematically under-nourishing ourselves. We need no-effort foods because the foods we're eating don't give us sustained nourishment…and without sustained nourishment, we don't have the energy needed to prepare the good foods our bodies do need! That's a seriously vicious cycle.

The good news is these addictions can be broken. Doing so does require some effort — nothing really good in life comes free — but the rewards of that effort dramatically outbalance the work.

Ditching no-good foods and eating the right stuff means more even, long-running energy, better moods and — yes! — improved, younger-looking skin.

THE **YOUNG SKIN** DIET

CALENDAR

THE YOUNG SKIN DIET CALENDAR

WEEK 1 | Prepare suggested foods as outlined. TYSD recipes are indicated in bold and are found in the Recipes section of this book.

Build Your Own Breakfast (**BYOB**) and Build Your Own Combo (**BYOC**) recipes are found in the BYOB and BYOC charts that follow the Calendars.

TYSD RECIPE	SATURDAY	SUNDAY	MONDAY
Morning Beverage	**Purifying Cinnamon Honey Tea**	1 cup tea (any) + lemon	**Stress Relief Black Tea with Lemon**
Breakfast	**No-More-Dark-Spots Oats**	BYOB	BYOB
Mid-Morning Snack	1 serving fruit (any) + 1 serving nuts/seeds (any)	1 serving fruit (any) + 1 serving nuts/seeds (any)	1 serving fruit (any) + 1 serving nuts/seeds (any)
Lunch	BYOC	**Repair-Your-Skin Thai Quinoa & Kale Salad**	
Afternoon Snack	1 serving fruit (any) + 1 serving nuts/seeds (any)	1 serving fruit (any) + 1 serving nuts/seeds (any)	1 serving fruit (any) + 1 serving nuts/seeds (any)
Dinner	**Omega-3 Garlic Barramundi with Mushrooms & Wild Rice**		**Tighten-Your-Skin Slow Cooker Yellow Curry**
Dessert	1 serving fruit (any)	1 serving fruit (any)	**Restorative Hot Honey Fruit**
Skin Treatment	**Skin-Brightening Coconut Oil Exfoliant**	**Calm Skin Turmeric Mask**	**Eliminate-Free-Radicals Olive Oil & Ginger Bath**

TIP Gray shading indicates when the suggested recipe yields multiple servings that are intended to be consumed over more than one day. Shaded boxes indicate the approximate number of days during which the recipe and its leftovers may be consumed. This may vary according to individual dietary needs.

Cooked dishes that yield more servings than the number of gray shaded days may be frozen and consumed at a later date in place of a BYOB or BYOC recipe.

TUESDAY	WEDNESDAY	THURSDAY	FRIDAY
1 cup tea (any) + lemon	**Anti-Aging Green Tea with Lemon**	1 cup tea (any) + lemon	**Restorative Ginger & Honey Tea**
Skin-Strengthening Veggie Egg Scramble	BYOB	BYOB	BYOB
1 serving fruit (any) + 1 serving nuts/seeds (any)	1 serving fruit (any) + 1 serving nuts/seeds (any)	1 serving fruit (any) + 1 serving nuts/seeds (any)	**Skin Plumping Berry Smoothie**
	Rejuvenating Mykonos Mediterranean Salad		BYOC
1 serving fruit (any) + 1 serving nuts/seeds (any)	**Collagen-Building Pomme Snack**	1 serving fruit (any) + 1 serving nuts/seeds (any)	1 serving fruit (any) + 1 serving nuts/seeds (any)
	1 serving fruit (any)	**Reverse-the-Clock Pistachio & Honey**	1 serving fruit (any)
Lemon Water & Cane Sugar Toning Mask	**No-More-Inflammation Honey & Olive Oil Mask**	**UV Damage Reducing Green Tea Mask**	**No-More-Irritation Cucumber Treatment**

THE YOUNG SKIN DIET CALENDAR

WEEK 2 | Prepare suggested foods as outlined. TYSD recipes are indicated in bold and are found in the Recipes section of this book.

Build Your Own Breakfast (**BYOB**) and Build Your Own Combo (**BYOC**) recipes are found in the BYOB and BYOC charts that follow the Calendars.

TYSD RECIPE	SATURDAY	SUNDAY	MONDAY
Morning Beverage	**Calming Rooibos Tea with Lemon**	1 cup tea (any) + lemon	**Anti-Inflammatory Chamomile Tea**
Breakfast	**BYOB**	**Powerhouse Quinoa**	
Mid-Morning Snack	1 serving fruit (any) + 1 serving nuts/seeds (any)	1 serving fruit (any) + 1 serving nuts/seeds (any)	**Healthy Skin Pistachio-Melon-Cherry Panache**
Lunch	**Skin Healing Kale with Lemon Vinaigrette**		
Afternoon Snack	1 serving fruit (any) + 1 serving nuts/seeds (any)	**Strong Skin Spinach & Chickpeas**	
Dinner	**The Ageless Ms. Fit Burger**		
Dessert	1 serving fruit (any)	**Cellular Repair Figs with Walnuts & Honey**	
Skin Treatment	**Skin-Brightening Coconut Oil Exfoliant**	**Calm Skin Turmeric Mask**	**Eliminate-Free-Radicals Olive Oil & Ginger Bath**

TIP Gray shading indicates when the suggested recipe yields multiple servings that are intended to be consumed over more than one day. Shaded boxes indicate the approximate number of days during which the recipe and its leftovers may be consumed. This may vary according to individual dietary needs.

Cooked dishes that yield more servings than the number of gray shaded days may be frozen and consumed at a later date in place of a BYOB or BYOC recipe.

TUESDAY	WEDNESDAY	THURSDAY	FRIDAY
1 cup tea (any) + lemon	**Clarifying Lemon-Ginger Water**	1 cup tea (any) + lemon	**Powerful Peppermint Tea**
		Procollagen Sweet Potato & Eggs	
	1 serving fruit (any) + 1 serving nuts/seeds (any)	1 serving fruit (any) + 1 serving nuts/seeds (any)	1 serving fruit (any) + 1 serving nuts/seeds (any)
	BYOC	**Stress-Fighting Salmon Cakes**	
	1 serving fruit (any) + 1 serving nuts/seeds (any)	1 serving fruit (any) + 1 serving nuts/seeds (any)	1 serving fruit (any) + 1 serving nuts/seeds (any)
Elasticity-Boost Asian Fusion Salad			
	Super Antioxidant Allspice Mango	1 serving fruit (any)	1 serving fruit (any)
Lemon Water & Cane Sugar Toning Mask	**No-More-Inflammation Honey & Olive Oil Mask**	**UV Damage Reducing Green Tea Mask**	**No-More-Irritation Cucumber Treatment**

THE YOUNG SKIN DIET CALENDAR

WEEK 3 | Prepare suggested foods as outlined. TYSD recipes are indicated in bold and are found in the Recipes section of this book.

Build Your Own Breakfast (**BYOB**) and Build Your Own Combo (**BYOC**) recipes are found in the BYOB and BYOC charts that follow the Calendars.

TYSD RECIPE	SATURDAY	SUNDAY	MONDAY
Morning Beverage	**Purifying Cinnamon Honey Tea**	1 cup tea (any) + lemon	**Stress Relief Black Tea with Lemon**
Breakfast	BYOB	**Photoaging Protection Quinoa & Vegetable Poached Eggs**	
Mid-Morning Snack	**Collagen-Boosting Strawberry-Melon Refresh**	1 serving fruit (any) + 1 serving nuts/seeds (any)	1 serving fruit (any) + 1 serving nuts/seeds (any)
Lunch	BYOC	**Smooth Skin Zucchini with Chicken**	
Afternoon Snack	**Revitalizing Goji Greatness**		
Dinner	**Tone 'n Texture Shrimp 'n Veggies**		
Dessert	1 serving fruit (any)	1 serving fruit (any)	**Sweet Dreams Smoothie**
Skin Treatment	**Skin-Brightening Coconut Oil Exfoliant**	**Calm Skin Turmeric Mask**	**Eliminate-Free-Radicals Olive Oil & Ginger Bath**

TIP Gray shading indicates when the suggested recipe yields multiple servings that are intended to be consumed over more than one day. Shaded boxes indicate the approximate number of days during which the recipe and its leftovers may be consumed. This may vary according to individual dietary needs.

Cooked dishes that yield more servings than the number of gray shaded days may be frozen and consumed at a later date in place of a BYOB or BYOC recipe.

TUESDAY	WEDNESDAY	THURSDAY	FRIDAY
1 cup tea (any) + lemon	**Anti-Aging Green Tea with Lemon**	1 cup tea (any) + lemon	**Restorative Ginger & Honey Tea**
BYOB	**Antioxidant Tropics Oats**	**BYOB**	**BYOB**
1 serving fruit (any) + 1 serving nuts/seeds (any)	1 serving fruit (any) + 1 serving nuts/seeds (any)	1 serving fruit (any) + 1 serving nuts/seeds (any)	1 serving fruit (any) + 1 serving nuts/seeds (any)
		BYOC	**BYOC**
	Hydrating Cucumber & Watermelon Cooldown	1 serving fruit (any) + 1 serving nuts/seeds (any)	1 serving fruit (any) + 1 serving nuts/seeds (any)
Anti-Wrinkle Spiced Salmon & Asparagus			
1 serving fruit (any)	1 serving fruit (any)	**Age-Defying Tropical Fruit Dessert**	1 serving fruit (any)
Lemon Water & Cane Sugar Toning Mask	**No-More-Inflammation Honey & Olive Oil Mask**	**UV Damage Reducing Green Tea Mask**	**No-More-Irritation Cucumber Treatment**

THE YOUNG SKIN DIET CALENDAR

WEEK 4 | Prepare suggested foods as outlined. TYSD recipes are indicated in bold and are found in the Recipes section of this book.

Build Your Own Breakfast (**BYOB**) and Build Your Own Combo (**BYOC**) recipes are found in the BYOB and BYOC charts that follow the Calendars.

TYSD RECIPE	SATURDAY	SUNDAY	MONDAY
Morning Beverage	**Calming Rooibos Tea with Lemon**	1 cup tea (any) + lemon	**Anti-Inflammatory Chamomile Tea**
Breakfast	BYOB	BYOB	BYOB
Mid-Morning Snack	1 serving fruit (any) + 1 serving nuts/seeds (any)	**Blemish Control Fruit Tea Cup**	
Lunch	**Young Skin Curry Soup**		
Afternoon Snack	1 serving fruit (any) + 1 serving nuts/seeds (any)	1 serving fruit (any) + 1 serving nuts/seeds (any)	1 serving fruit (any) + 1 serving nuts/seeds (any)
Dinner	BYOC	**Erase-the-Photodamage Pretty Powerful Pasta**	
Dessert	1 serving fruit (any)	1 serving fruit (any)	**UV Protection Citrus Salad**
Skin Treatment	**Skin-Brightening Coconut Oil Exfoliant**	**Calm Skin Turmeric Mask**	**Eliminate-Free-Radicals Olive Oil & Ginger Bath**

TIP Gray shading indicates when the suggested recipe yields multiple servings that are intended to be consumed over more than one day. Shaded boxes indicate the approximate number of days during which the recipe and its leftovers may be consumed. This may vary according to individual dietary needs.

Cooked dishes that yield more servings than the number of gray shaded days may be frozen and consumed at a later date in place of a BYOB or BYOC recipe.

TUESDAY	WEDNESDAY	THURSDAY	FRIDAY
1 cup tea (any) + lemon	**Clarifying Lemon-Ginger Water**	1 cup tea (any) + lemon	**Powerful Peppermint Tea**
Make-Your-Skin-Glow Spinach & Eggs	BYOB	BYOB	**Natural Sunscreen Green Eggs & Omegas**
1 serving fruit (any) + 1 serving nuts/seeds (any)	1 serving fruit (any) + 1 serving nuts/seeds (any)	1 serving fruit (any) + 1 serving nuts/seeds (any)	1 serving fruit (any) + 1 serving nuts/seeds (any)
	BYOC	BYOC	BYOC
1 serving fruit (any) + 1 serving nuts/seeds (any)	1 serving fruit (any) + 1 serving nuts/seeds (any)	**Radiant Skin Red Fruit Medley**	1 serving fruit (any) + 1 serving nuts/seeds (any)
BYOC	BYOC	BYOC	BYOC
	1 serving fruit (any)	1 serving fruit (any)	1 serving fruit (any)
Lemon Water & Cane Sugar Toning Mask	**No-More-Inflammation Honey & Olive Oil Mask**	**UV Damage Reducing Green Tea Mask**	**No-More-Irritation Cucumber Treatment**

THE **YOUNG SKIN** DIET

BUILD YOUR OWN
BREAKFAST GUIDE

BUILD YOUR OWN BREAKFAST (BYOB)

ROLLED OATS BASE
½ cup gluten free rolled oats, dry

2 tsp. unrefined coconut oil, softened

1 tsp. chia seeds

1 tsp. honey

Stir rolled oats base ingredients together in a small bowl.

Choose TYSD COMBO 1, 2 or 3. Top oat base with selected TYSD TOPPINGS, stir, and enjoy!

Each rolled oats TYSD COMBO makes 1 serving.

TIP No need to cook oats or use milk. These combos can be enjoyed dry.

TYSD COMBO	TYSD TOPPING 1	TYSD TOPPING 2	TYSD TOPPING 3	TYSD TOPPING 4
1	5 cashews, roughly chopped	¼ cup goji berries	¼ tsp. cinnamon	dash of salt
2	5-10 walnuts, roughly chopped	1 date, pitted & chopped	½ apple, diced	½ tbsp. coconut flakes
3	5 walnuts, roughly chopped	15 blueberries	2 tbsp. pomegranate seeds	¼ tsp. cinnamon

OAT BRAN BASE
⅔ cup oat bran, dry

2 cups water

¼ tsp. salt

Prepare oat bran according to package instructions, using water (add salt if desired).

Choose TYSD COMBO 1, 2 or 3. Stir selected TYSD TOPPINGS into oat bran while cooking. Enjoy!

Each oat bran TYSD COMBO **makes 2 servings.**

TIP Refrigerate leftovers. To reheat, cook in microwave on high for 1 to 2 minutes. Stir. Serve.

TYSD COMBO	TYSD TOPPING 1	TYSD TOPPING 2	TYSD TOPPING 3	TYSD TOPPING 4
1	1 date, pitted and chopped	1 tsp. honey	¼ tsp. cinnamon	6 walnuts, chopped
2	2 tbsp. raisins	1 tsp. honey	¼ tsp. cinnamon	2 tsp. coconut oil
3	½ banana, chopped	1 tsp. honey	2 tsp. coconut oil	6 walnuts, chopped

12 RECIPES. READY IN 15 MINUTES OR LESS.

Choose TYSD COMBO 1, 2 or 3.

Heat olive oil over medium heat in a non-stick skillet. Briefly heat selected TYSD SPICES in skillet. For TYSD COMBO 1, heat tomatoes with spices.

Scramble eggs in skillet until cooked through. Serve with selected TYSD SIDE. Each egg TYSD COMBO makes 1 serving.

EGG BASE
2 eggs

1 tsp. extra virgin olive oil

TYSD COMBO	TYSD SPICE 1	TYSD SPICE 2	TYSD SPICE 3	TYSD SIDE
1	½ tsp. rosemary	ground black pepper, to taste	¼ tsp. turmeric	Sliced tomato, heated in skillet
2	¼ tsp. turmeric	ground black pepper, to taste	⅛ tsp. sea salt	¼ cup oats, top with honey & cinnamon
3	¼ tsp. oregano	ground black pepper, to taste	⅛ tsp. sea salt	½ cup watermelon, chilled & cubed

Prepare quinoa in water according to package instructions.

Choose TYSD COMBO 1, 2 or 3. Stir selected TYSD TOPPINGS into quinoa when finished cooking.

Each quinoa TYSD COMBO **makes 2 servings**.

TIP *For TYSD COMBO 1, add cinnamon sticks to quinoa while cooking.

QUINOA BASE
½ cup quinoa, dry

1 cup water

TYSD COMBO	TYSD TOPPING 1	TYSD TOPPING 2	TYSD TOPPING 3	TYSD TOPPING 4
1	2 tsp. honey	½ tsp. coarsely ground salt	6 walnuts, chopped	2 cinnamon sticks*
2	½ cup strawberries, sliced	½ cup banana, sliced	2 tsp. coconut oil	1 tsp. honey or rice milk
3	2 tbsp. pumpkin seeds	¼ cup dried cranberries	1 tsp. cinnamon + dash of salt	2 tsp. honey + 1 tsp. coconut oil

THE **YOUNG SKIN** DIET

BUILD YOUR OWN COMBO GUIDE

BUILD YOUR OWN COMBO (BYOC)

SALAD BASE | Choose TYSD COMBO 1, 2 or 3.

Vigorously mix selected TYSD DRESSING ingredients.

Place selected TYSD SALAD BASE in bowl. Toss with dressing, top with selected TYSD TOPPINGS and serve.

Each salad TYSD COMBO **makes 2 servings**.

NOTE EVOO means Extra Virgin Olive Oil.

TYSD COMBO	TYSD SALAD BASE	TYSD TOPPING 1	TYSD TOPPING 2	TYSD TOPPING 3	TYSD DRESSING
1	5 oz. baby spring mix lettuce	4 poached eggs	¼ cup sun-dried tomatoes	½ cup. kalamata olives	2 tbsp. EVOO + 1½ tbsp. red wine vinegar + ½ tsp. dijon mustard + salt & pepper, to taste
2	5 oz. baby spring mix lettuce	1 sweet potato, cubed and roasted (to roast, toss with EVOO + dash salt & ground black pepper; bake at 400 degrees for 20 min.)	¼ cup dried cranberries	¼ cup candied pecans	1 tbsp. dijon mustard + 2 tbsp. red wine vinegar + 1 tsp. honey + ⅓ cup EVOO
3	5 oz. butter lettuce	½ cup black beans	½ avocado, thinly sliced	1 tomato, diced	2 tbsp. fresh-squeezed lime juice + 2 tbsp. EVOO + 1 garlic clove, minced + ½ tsp. honey + ½ tsp. salt + ⅛ tsp. coriander + 1 tbsp. cilantro, chopped + ½ tsp. jalapeno pepper, chopped

13 RECIPES. 15 MINUTES OR LESS ACTIVE PREP.

Choose TYSD COMBO 1, 2 or 3.

Prepare selected TYSD GRAIN BASE according to package instructions. For quinoa, use low-sodium vegetable broth in place of water. Stir in selected TYSD TOPPINGS and SEASONING. Serve.

Each whole grain TYSD COMBO **makes 4 servings**.

NOTE EVOO means Extra Virgin Olive Oil.

WHOLE GRAIN BASE

TYSD COMBO	TYSD GRAIN BASE	TYSD TOPPING 1	TYSD TOPPING 2	TYSD TOPPING 3	TYSD SEASONING
1	1 cup organic white quinoa, dry	15 oz. black beans, drained & rinsed	1 red pepper + 1 red onion + 3 garlic cloves, diced and sauteed in EVOO	1 avocado, peeled and cubed	2 tbsp. cumin + salt & ground black pepper, to taste
2	1 cup wild rice, dry	1½ cups red grapes, halved	1 cup roasted unsalted cashews	3 stalks green onion, chopped	Vinaigrette = 4 tbsp. EVOO + 1 tbsp. fresh-squeezed lemon juice + 2 tbsp. white balsamic vinegar + 1 tbsp. honey + 1 garlic clove, crushed + salt, to taste (mix vigorously)
3	1 cup organic white quinoa, dry	1 red onion + 1 garlic clove, diced and sauteed in EVOO	1 cup pumpkin puree, heated in skillet with onion and garlic	2 cups baby spinach leaves, stirred into hot quinoa until just wilted	salt + ground black pepper + hazelnuts, to taste

BUILD YOUR OWN COMBO (BYOC)

SLOW COOKER | Choose TYSD COMBO 1, 2 or 3.

Place selected TYSD SLOW COOKER BASE IN-GREDIENTS in crock pot.

Add selected TYSD SEASONINGS, stir and cook on low for specified time.

Each slow cooker TYSD COMBO **makes 6 to 8 servings**.

NOTE *For TYSD COMBO 1, add hazelnuts just before serving.

TYSD COMBO	TYSD SLOW COOKER BASE INGREDIENTS
1	1 butternut squash, peeled, seeded and chopped into 1-inch cubes + 1 yellow onion, peeled and chopped + 3 carrots, chopped + 1 fuji or red delicious apple, chopped with skin on + 14 oz. low-sodium vegetable broth (Cook for 6 hours.)
2	3 cups full fat coconut milk + 2 cups low-sodium vegetable broth + 2 cups dry arborio rice + 2 cups chicken, cubed + 1½ cups carrots, sliced (Cook for 4 hours. Add peas and cook for 30 more minutes.)
3	1 red onion, thinly sliced + 4 cups low-sodium vegetable broth + 14 oz. full fat coconut milk (or coconut cream) + 5 cups collard greens + 1 lb. sweet potatoes, cubed (Cook for 4 hours.)

13 RECIPES. 15 MINUTES OR LESS ACTIVE PREP.

TYSD SEASONING 1	TYSD SEASONING 2	TYSD SEASONING 3	TYSD SEASONING 4	TYSD SEASONING 5
½ tsp. cinnamon	¼ tsp. nutmeg	2 tbsp. honey	¼ cup toasted hazelnuts*	salt + ground black pepper, to taste
2 tbsp. curry powder	1 tbsp. lime juice	½ tsp. ground black pepper	cayenne pepper, to taste	1 cup peas
1 garlic clove, crushed	1 tbsp. ginger, grated	salt, to taste	ground black pepper, to taste	dash of cinnamon

BUILD YOUR OWN COMBO (BYOC)

PROTEIN BASE | Choose TYSD COMBO 1 or 2.

Mix selected TYSD MARINADE ingredients together. Marinate selected TYSD PROTEIN BASE for 4 or more hours.

Follow TYSD SIMPLE INSTRUCTIONS for cooking. Serve with selected TYSD SIDES.

Each protein TYSD COMBO **makes 4 servings**.

TYSD COMBO	TYSD PROTEIN BASE	TYSD MARINADE 1	TYSD MARINADE 2	TYSD MARINADE 3	TYSD MARINADE 4
1	1 lb. free-range chicken breasts or thighs	½ cup EVOO	⅛ cup fresh-squeezed lemon juice	3 garlic cloves, minced	1½ tsp. salt + ¼ tsp. ground black pepper
2	1 lb. wild-caught shrimp	½ cup EVOO	⅛ cup fresh-squeezed lemon juice	3 garlic cloves, minced	1½ tsp. salt + ¼ tsp. ground black pepper

PROTEIN BASE | Choose TYSD COMBO 1 or 2.

Mix selected TYSD SPICE ingredients together. Coat selected TYSD PROTEIN BASE in TYSD COOKING OIL. Season to taste with spice mix.

Follow TYSD SIMPLE INSTRUCTIONS for cooking. Serve with selected TYSD SIDES.

Each protein TYSD COMBO **makes 4 servings**.

TYSD COMBO	TYSD PROTEIN BASE	TYSD SPICE 1	TYSD SPICE 2	TYSD SPICE 3	TYSD SPICE 4
1	1 lb. free-range chicken thighs	1 tsp. oregano	1 tsp. cumin	½ tsp. ground black pepper	¼ tsp. salt
2	1 lb. wild-caught salmon	1 tsp. kosher salt + 1 tsp. ground black pepper	½ tsp. cumin	½ tsp. coriander	½ tsp. allspice

13 RECIPES. 15 MINUTES OR LESS ACTIVE PREP.

NOTE EVOO means Extra Virgin Olive Oil.

TYSD MARINADE 5	TYSD SIDE 1	TYSD SIDE 2	TYSD SIMPLE INSTRUCTIONS
1½ tsp. honey	1 cup wild rice	1 lb. steamed broccoli	Bake marinated chicken in glass baking dish at 425 degrees for 45 minutes.
1½ tsp. honey	1 cup wild rice	1 lb. steamed green beans	Saute marinated shrimp over medium heat until cooked through, about 3 to 5 minutes.

NOTE EVOO means Extra Virgin Olive Oil.

TYSD COOKING OIL	TYSD SIDE 1	TYSD SIDE 2	TYSD SIMPLE INSTRUCTIONS
2 tsp. EVOO	Baked sweet potatoes topped with coconut oil and cinnamon	1 lb. steamed brussels sprouts	Bake seasoned chicken in glass baking dish at 425 degrees for 45 minutes.
2 tsp. EVOO	Baked Stokes purple sweet potatoes topped with coconut oil and cinnamon	1 lb. poached asparagus	Bake seasoned salmon in foil-lined baking sheet at 400 degrees for 20 minutes.

THE **YOUNG SKIN** DIET

MORNING BEVERAGES

CLARIFYING LEMON-GINGER WATER

1 cup filtered water

Bring water to a boil.

1 tbsp. fresh-squeezed lemon juice + ¼ tsp. lemon zest

Steep ginger in water for 3 minutes.

If not using a tea steeper for ginger, strain ginger from water and pour water into mug. Add lemon juice and zest. Stir. Enjoy!

1 tbsp. ginger, minced or grated

TIP After consuming lemon-ginger water, rinse mouth with regular water to protect tooth enamel.

SCIENCE & NUTRITION

Lemon Juice + Lemon Zest: Vitamin C, beta-carotene, flavonoids, limonene and folic acid collectively provide the body with antioxidant, antimicrobial and anti-carcinogenic benefits that improve skin health. The micronutrients in lemon's juice and zest work synergistically to compound the antioxidant benefits for skin.

- *Silalahi, J. "Anticancer and health protective properties of citrus fruit components," Asia Pacific Journal of Clinical Nutrition. 2002 Mar.; 11(1): 79-84.*
- *Crowell, P. and M. Gould. "Chemoprevention and therapy of cancer by d-limonene," Critical Reviews in Oncogenesis. 1994; 5(1): 1-22.*

Ginger: The phytochemistry of ginger provides powerful anti-inflammatory and antioxidative effects as well as improved blood circulation. Enhanced blood circulation through capillaries feeding skin's inner layers and young cells enables skin cells to be healthier throughout their lifecycle as they move outward to the skin's surface.

- *Shokri Mashhadi, N., et al. "Anti-oxidative and anti-inflammatory effects of ginger in health and physical activity: review of current evidence," International Journal of Preventive Medicine. 2013 Apr.; 4(Supp. 1): S36-S42.*

10 calories; 0g fat; 0g sat. fat; 0mg cholesterol; 0mg sodium; 40mg potassium; 3g carbohydrates; 0g fiber; 1g sugar; 0g protein. 1 serving.

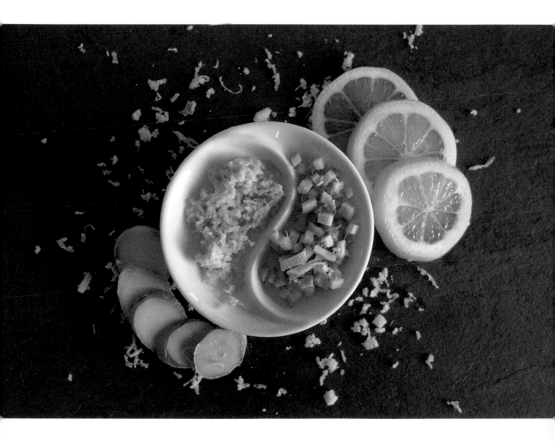

ANTI-INFLAMMATORY CHAMOMILE TEA

1 cup filtered water	Prepare tea according to package instructions.
1 sachet chamomile tea	Squeeze lemon juice into tea, stir and serve.
Juice from ¼ lemon	

SCIENCE & NUTRITION

Chamomile: Polyphenols in chamomile are effective anti-inflammatories that can help promote cellular health in skin and elsewhere. The calming effect on inflammation allows skin's biological processes, including normal cellular function and healing, to work more efficiently and thus clear impurities and damage from skin at an accelerated rate.

- *Bhaskaran, N., et al. "Chamomile: an anti-inflammatory agent inhibits inducible nitric oxide synthase expression by blocking RelA/p65 activity," International Journal of Molecular Medicine. 2010 Dec.; 26(6): 935-940.*

- *Drummond, E.M., et al. "Inhibition of proinflammatory biomarkers in THP1 macrophages by polyphenols derived from chamomile, meadowsweet and willow bark," Phytotherapy Research. 2013 Apr.; 27(4): 588-594.*

5 calories; 0g fat; 0g sat. fat; 0mg cholesterol; 0mg sodium; 20mg potassium; 1g carbohydrates; 0g fiber; 1g sugar; 0g protein. 1 serving.

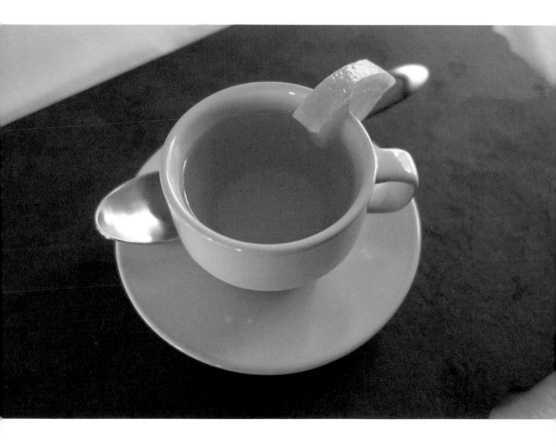

ANTI-AGING GREEN TEA WITH LEMON

1 cup filtered water | Prepare tea according to package instructions.

1 sachet green tea | Squeeze lemon juice into tea, stir and serve.

Juice from ¼ lemon

SCIENCE & NUTRITION

Green Tea + Lemon Juice: Potent antioxidants in green tea known as catechins counteract oxidative stress and the signs of aging on skin. Lemon juice and its high levels of vitamin C protect catechins in the body and enable 500% greater absorption.

- *Green, R., et al. "Common tea formulations modulate in vitro digestive recovery of green tea catechins," Molecular Nutrition and Food Research. 2007 Sep.; 51(9): 1152-1162.*

Green Tea: The caffeine in green tea helps the body slough skin cells damaged by UV rays, thus negating some sun damage and revealing healthy skin.

- *Heffernan, T., et al. "ATR-Chk1 pathway inhibition promotes apoptosis after UV treatment in primary human keratinocytes: potential basis for the UV protective effects of caffeine," Journal of Investigative Dermatology. 2009; 129: 1805-1815.*

5 calories; 0g fat; 0g sat. fat; 0mg cholesterol; 0mg sodium; 20mg potassium; 1g carbohydrates; 0g fiber; 1g sugar; 0g protein. 1 serving.

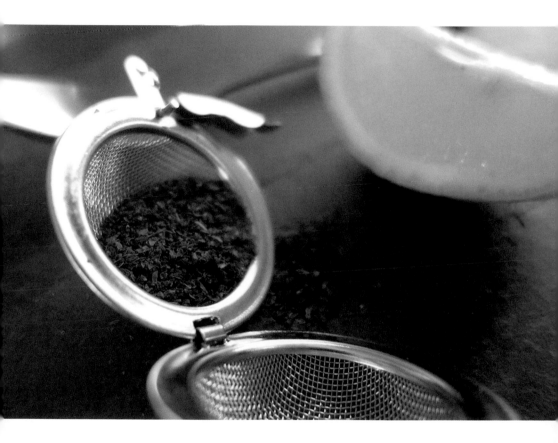

CALMING ROOIBOS TEA WITH LEMON

1 cup filtered water

1 sachet rooibos tea

Juice from ¼ lemon

Prepare tea according to package instructions.

Squeeze lemon juice into tea, stir and serve.

SCIENCE & NUTRITION

Rooibos Tea: Among its many antioxidants, rooibos offers aspalathin, which is not known to be found in any other foods. Aspalathin and polyphenols from rooibos tea suppress inflammation and oxidation in many of the body's systems and reduce production of cortisol, the so-called stress hormone. Since cortisol is known to cause excessive oil production, rooibos tea helps maintain even skin complexion and tone, for a collected and youthful appearance.

- *Schloms, L., et al. "The influence of aspalathus linearis (rooibos) and dihydrochalcones on adrenal steroidogenesis: quantification of steroid intermediates and end products in H295R cells," The Journal of Steroid Biochemistry and Molecular Biology. 2012 Feb.; 128(3-5): 128-138.*

- *Talbott, S. Cortisol Control and the Beauty Connection. Ch. 4: "Inside-out help for wrinkles, acne, and 'problem' skin," Hunter House Publishers, Inc., 2007.*

Rooibos Tea + Lemon: The antioxidant profile of rooibos tea, including the aspalathin flavonoid, is effective at calming the body's systems, reducing inflammation and warding off infection, all of which benefits the skin. Lemon helps tea's antioxidants remain potent in the body.

- *Joubert, E. and D. Ferreira. "Antioxidants of rooibos tea – a possible explanation for its health promoting properties?" The SA Journal of Food Science and Nutrition. 1996; 8(3): 79-83.*

5 calories; 0g fat; 0g sat. fat; 0mg cholesterol; 0mg sodium; 20mg potassium; 1g carbohydrates; 0g fiber; 1g sugar; 0g protein. 1 serving.

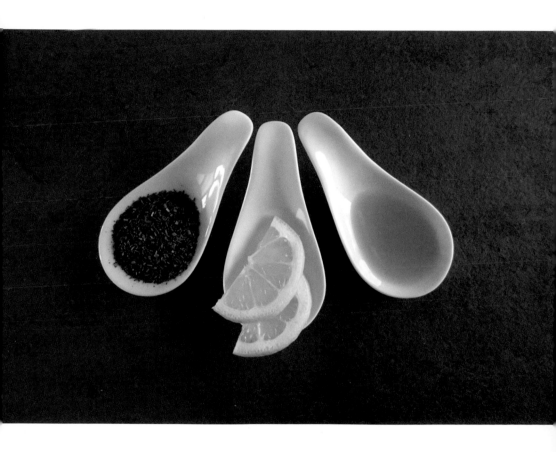

RESTORATIVE GINGER & HONEY TEA

1 cup filtered water	Bring water to a boil.
1 tbsp. ginger, minced	Steep ginger in water for 3 minutes. If not using a tea steeper for ginger, strain ginger from water and pour water into mug.
1 tbsp. honey	
	Add honey, stir and drink.

SCIENCE & NUTRITION

Ginger + Honey: Synergistic antibacterial and antimicrobial effects from ginger and honey have been clinically demonstrated to enhance the foods' protective and restorative effects on health. Combating infection and microbial presence in the skin allows skin's natural complexion to overcome inflammation, redness and proneness to breakouts

- *Aruna G., et al. "Combined effect of ginger and honey against salmonellosis," Global Journal for Research Analysis. 2014 Aug.; 3(8): 1-3.*

60 calories; 0g fat; 0g sat. fat; 0mg cholesterol; 0mg sodium; 10mg potassium; 17g carbohydrates; 0g fiber; 16g sugar; 0g protein. 1 serving.

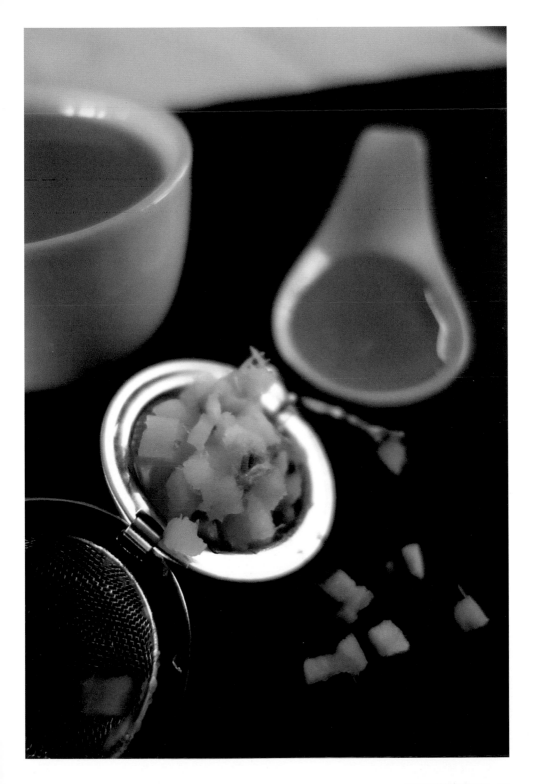

PURIFYING CINNAMON-HONEY TEA

1 cup filtered water	Bring water to a boil.
¼ tsp. cinnamon	Pour water into a large mug. Add cinnamon and stir. Add honey, stir again and drink.
1 tbsp. honey	

SCIENCE & NUTRITION

Cinnamon + Honey: Honey's antimicrobial and anti-inflammatory effects alone are potent, and cinnamon and honey exhibit additive and synergistic qualities in reducing infectious agents and cellular inflammation, thereby purifying the skin's ecosystem more rapidly. Additionally, cinnamon has positive effects on the glucose/insulin system and can help mitigate sugar-related blood pressure elevations that might otherwise present with honey consumption. Cinnamon and honey work together to enable antimicrobial and anti-inflammatory bene-fits with reductions in sugar-related drawbacks.

- *Preuss, H.G., et al. "Whole cinnamon and aqueous extracts ameliorate sucrose-in-duced blood pressure elevations in spontaneously hypertensive rats," Journal of the American College of Nutrition. 2006; 25(2): 144-150.*

60 calories; 0g fat; 0g sat. fat; 0mg cholesterol; 0mg sodium; 10mg potassium; 17g carbohydrates; 0g fiber; 16g sugar; 0g protein. 1 serving.

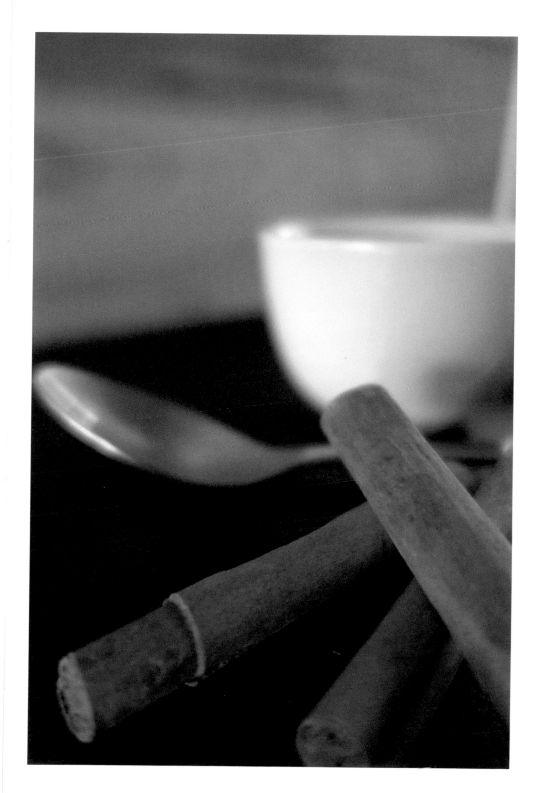

ANTI-OXIDANT TROPICS OATS

½ **cup gluten-free rolled oats**

1 **cup water**

¼ **Fuji or Red Delicious apple, diced**

1 **date, pit removed and chopped**

1 **tsp. honey**

1 **tsp. orange juice**

2 to 3 **walnuts, chopped**

1 **tbsp. unsweetened coconut flakes**

½ **tbsp. unrefined coconut oil**

¼ **tsp. chia seeds**

Prepare oats according to package instructions, using water.

When oatmeal is cooked, add apple, date, honey, orange juice, walnuts, coconut flakes, coconut oil, and chia seeds. Stir. Serve.

SCIENCE & NUTRITION

Chia Seeds: Chia seeds have been noted for their high concentration of antioxidants, including phenolic acids and isoflavones called caffeic acid, gallic acid and daidzin, all of which help ward off and reverse oxidative damage in the skin stemming from metabolic activity, stressors and environmental factors.

- *Martinez-Cruz, O., et al. "Phytochemical profile and nutraceutical potential of chia seeds (salvia hispanica l.) by liquid chromatography," Journal of Chromatography A. 2014 Jun.; 1346: 43-48.*

Oats: The beta-glucans found in oats provide immune system strengthening effects, including that which helps cells control growth and metabolic action in the skin. This helps to clear the skin and maintain a healthy complexion.

- *Akramiene, D., et al. "Effects of beta-glucans on the immune system," Medicina. 2007; 43(8): 597-606.*
- *Tsikitis, V., et al. "Beta-glucan affects leukocyte navigation in a complex chemotactic gradient," Surgery. 2004 Aug.; 136(2): 384-389.*

Dates: Tannins, which are found in dates, have been associated with antimicrobial, anticarcinogenic, antimutagenic, and antioxidant activity, as well as reduced blood pressure. These effects collectively improve skin quality by fighting factors that contribute to skin aging and skin-based disease.

- *Chung, K., et al. "Tannins and human health: a review," Critical Reviews in Food Science and Nutrition. 1998 Aug.; 38(6): 421-464.*

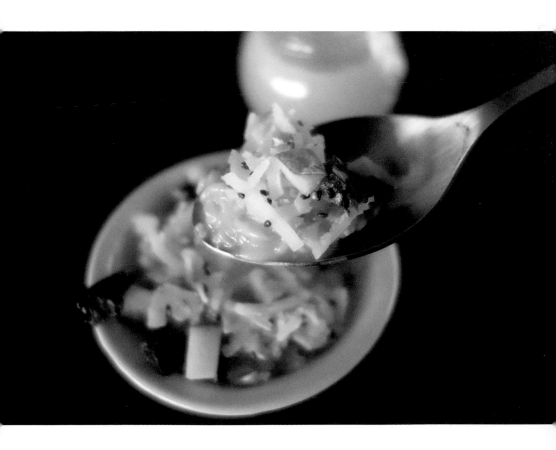

480 calories; 21g fat; 11g sat. fat; 0mg cholesterol; 60mg sodium; 270mg potassium; 71g carbohydrates; 9g fiber; 33g sugar; 8g protein. 1 serving.

PROCOLLAGEN SWEET POTATO & EGGS

1 large sweet potato, sliced into ¾-inch wedges with skin left on

1 tbsp. unrefined coconut oil, melted

1 tsp. turmeric

1 tsp. ground black pepper

Dash sea salt + 1 tsp. for poaching eggs

Dash cayenne pepper

4 eggs (with Omega-3s), chilled

2 tsp. white wine vinegar

8 oz. orange juice

Preheat oven to 450. Place potato wedges in glass baking dish and toss with 1 tbsp. melted coconut oil. Add turmeric and black pepper. Season with sea salt and cayenne pepper to taste. Toss to coat evenly. Bake wedges for 25 to 30 minutes. When potatoes are finished cooking, remove from oven and place on serving plates.

While potatoes bake, fill a large, deep non-stick skillet with 1½ inches of water and heat over medium heat. Stir in vinegar and 1 tsp. salt. While water heats, crack each egg into a separate ramekin and set aside.

Once vinegar water reaches simmer, slowly lower ramekins into water, allowing eggs to enter water. Do not agitate the egg whites or they will feather. Turn off heat, cover and let eggs poach for 5 minutes. Do not disturb eggs while poaching. Meanwhile, line a plate with paper towels.

Remove eggs from water with a slotted spoon and place on paper towel lined plate to drain water.

Place cooked eggs atop potato wedges. Sprinkle with turmeric, ground pepper, sea salt, and cayenne pepper. Serve. To eat, break eggs and toss potato wedges in yolk. Serve orange juice as beverage.

TIP Poached eggs may be stored in ice water overnight in fridge and reheated the next day by placing them in heated water (about 140 degrees) for 2 minutes.

SCIENCE & NUTRITION

Turmeric + Black Pepper: Potent anti-inflammatory and pro-metabolic benefits are derived from the curcumin and curcuminoids found in turmeric. The piperine in black pepper enhances the bioavailiability of curcumin by 2,000%. Curcumin has been shown to interact with collagen to enhance dermal repair and reduce scarring.

- *Shoba, G., et al. "Influence of piperine on the pharmacokinetics of curcumin in animals and human volunteers," Planta Medica. 1998 May; 64(4): 353-356.*

- *Panchatcharam, M., et al. "Curcumin improves wound healing by modulating collagen and decreasing reactive oxygen species," Molecular and Cellular Biochemistry. 2006 Mar.; 290(1): 87-96.*

Eggs + Orange Juice: Collagen-building lysine and proline amino acids are found in egg whites, while yolks provide Omega-3 fatty acids that reduce inflammation and help biological processes like collagen formation occur more efficiently. Vitamin C from orange juice binds with lysine and proline to form procollagen, which the body uses directly in the manufacture of collagen.

- *English, J., et al. "The collagen connection," Nutrition Review. 2013 Apr.*

Sweet Potatoes + Coconut Oil: Vitamin A, which is abundant in sweet potatoes, provides antioxidant benefits in the skin by protecting and rebuilding collagen. The fats in coconut oil help the body metabolize Vitamin A.

- *Varani, J., et al. "Vitamin A antagonizes decreased cell growth and elevated collagen-degrading matrix metalloproteinases and stimulates collagen accumulation in naturally aged human skin," Journal of Investigative Dermatology. 2000 Mar.; 114(3): 480-486.*

310 calories; 16g fat; 9g sat. fat; 430mg cholesterol; 220mg sodium; 590mg potassium; 28g carbohydrates; 2g fiber; 13g sugar; 14g protein. 2 servings. Excludes orange juice.

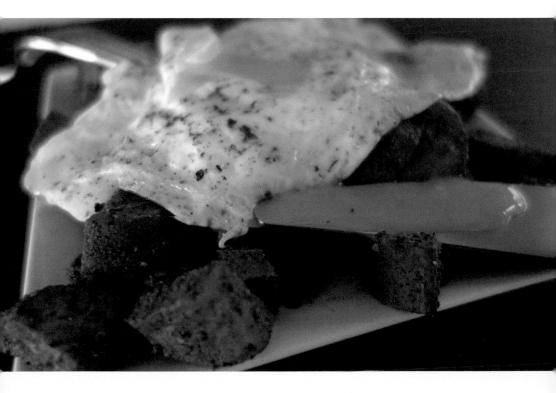

SKIN-STRENGTHENING VEGGIE EGG SCRAMBLE

2 eggs, beaten	Fill a small non-stick skillet 1 centimeter deep with water and bring to a boil. Meanwhile, beat eggs in a medium bowl and set aside.
4 broccoli florets, chopped into bite-size pieces	
3 mini heirloom tomatoes, halved	Once water reaches boil, add broccoli, cover, and heat for 3 minutes. Remove from heat and drain.
2 tsp. super sweet mini bell peppers, finely chopped	Add broccoli, tomatoes, and peppers to eggs. Season to taste with oregano, salt, pepper, and cayenne. Lightly stir egg mixture to combine ingredients.
Oregano	Return skillet to stovetop and heat over medium-high. Add just enough olive oil to lightly coat bottom of skillet. Once olive oil is heated, swirl to coat bottom of skillet evenly. Add egg mixture and scramble until eggs start to cook. Turn heat down to medium or medium-low to keep eggs fluffy and prevent burning. Continue cooking until eggs are heated through.
Sea salt	
Ground black pepper	
Cayenne pepper	
Extra virgin olive oil	

SCIENCE & NUTRITION

Egg: Providing EPA and DHA Omega-3 fatty acids, along with high bio-availability protein (and negligible effects on blood cholesterol), eggs offer important macronutrients and micronutrients for skin health. Proteins contribute amino acids for production of the body's collagen, elastin and keratin protein structures in the skin; Omega-3 fats lubricate cell components and provide volume to the subcutaneous lipid layer; and egg yolk provides carotenoid antioxidants.

- *Riedeger, N., et al. "A systemic review of the roles of n-3 fatty acids in health and disease," Journal of the American Dietetic Association. 2009 Apr.; 109(4): 668-679.*
- *Applegate, E. "Introduction: nutritional and functional roles of eggs in the diet," Journal of the American College of Nutrition. 2000; 19(Supp. 5): 495S-498S.*

Cayenne Pepper + Black Pepper: Spices contain high concentrations of antioxidants without contributing to daily caloric, fat, sugar or carbohydrate intake, offering an efficient source of antioxidants to complement meals.

- *Suhaj, M. "Spice antioxidants isolation and their antiradical activity: a review," Journal of Food Composition and Analysis. 2006 Sep.-Nov.; 19(6-7): 531-537.*

Broccoli: Among the 27 vegetables most commonly consumed in the United States, broccoli has the highest cellular antioxidant activity. Broccoli's antioxidants contribute to reductions in cellular oxidative stress and thereby slow processes that contribute to skin aging.

- *Song, W., et al. "Cellular antioxidant activity of common vegetables," Journal of Agricultural and Food Chemistry. 2010; 58(11): 6621-6629.*

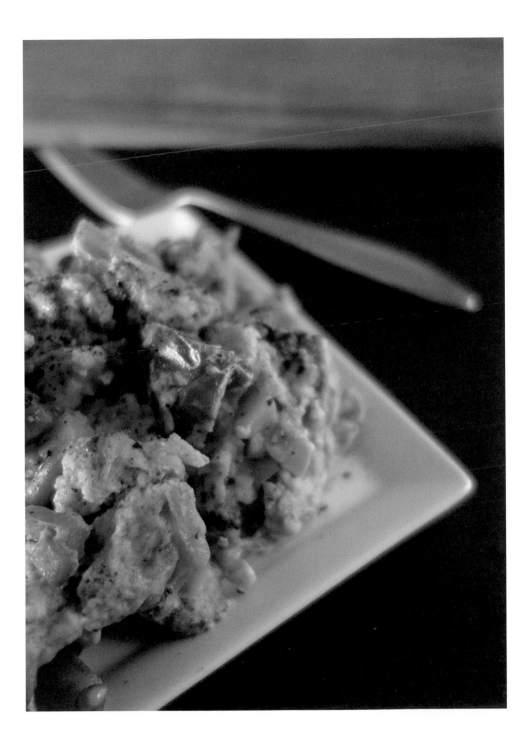

220 calories; 14g fat; 4g sat. fat; 430mg cholesterol; 370mg sodium; 500mg potassium; 11g carbohydrates; 1g fiber; 5g sugar; 14g protein. 1 serving.

POWERHOUSE QUINOA

1 cup dry white quinoa

2 cups water

1 Fuji, Red Delicious or Gala apple, cored and thinly sliced

¼ tsp. cinnamon

Sea salt

½ tbsp. honey

¼ to ½ cup chopped pistachios

¼ cup goji berries

Low fat coconut milk

Mix quinoa, water, apple slices, cinnamon, and a dash of salt in pot. Bring to a boil. Reduce heat, cover, and simmer for 15 minutes or until water is absorbed.

Remove from heat. Stir in honey. Serve and top with chopped pistachios and goji berries. Stir in desired amount of coconut milk.

SCIENCE & NUTRITION

Organic Quinoa: Studies indicate that organic crops, including fruits, vegetables and grains, contain higher levels of desirable minerals and vitamins and lower levels of nitrates and other undesirable elements. Consuming organic quinoa maximizes this food's positive effects on health and the skin, while reducing exposure to chemicals from foods that can reduce the body's resilience to environmental and age-related stressors that erode skin's youthfulness.

- *Worthington, V. "Nutritional quality of organic versus conventional fruits, vegetables, and grains," The Journal of Alternative and Complementary Medicine. 2001 Apr.; 7(2): 161-173.*

- *Huber, M., et al. "Organic food and impact on human health: assessing the status quo and prospects of research," NJAS-Wageningen Journal of Life Sciences. 2011 Dec.; 58(3-4): 103-109.*

Pistachios: Ranking among the top 50 foods with antioxidant capabilities, pistachios contain a host of phenolic compounds that fight inflammation and free radicals, the effects of which include healthier, younger-looking skin.

- *Tomaino, A., et al. "Antioxidant activity and phenolic profile of pistachio (pistacia vera l., variety bronte) seeds and skins," Biochimie. 2010 Sep.; 92(9): 1115-1122.*

300 calories; 7g fat; 1g sat. fat; 0mg cholesterol; 100mg sodium; 280mg potassium; 52g carbohydrates; 7g fiber; 17g sugar; 10g protein. 4 servings.

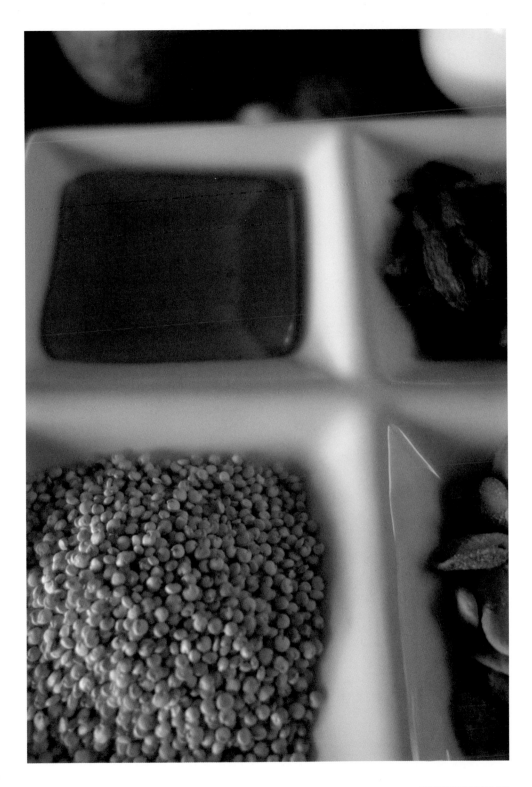

PHOTOAGING PROTECTION QUINOA & VEGETABLE POACHED EGGS

2 tsp. white wine vinegar

1 tsp. sea salt

2 eggs, chilled

Handful of baby romaine lettuce leaves

½ avocado, diced

½ cup dry red quinoa, prepared according to package instructions

4 asparagus spears, steamed and chopped into 2-inch long pieces

3 mini heirloom tomatoes, halved

2 tbsp. chopped walnuts

Ground black pepper

Turmeric

Extra virgin olive oil

Fill a large, deep non-stick skillet with 1½ inches of water and heat over medium heat. Stir in vinegar and salt. While water heats, crack each egg into a separate ramekin and set aside.

Once vinegar water reaches simmer, slowly lower ramekins into water, allowing eggs to enter water. Do not agitate the egg whites or they will feather. Turn off heat, cover and let eggs poach for 5 minutes. Do not disturb eggs while poaching. Meanwhile, line a plate with paper towels.

Remove eggs from water with a slotted spoon and place on paper towel lined plate to drain water.

Place lettuce leaves in a bowl. Top with avocado, quinoa, asparagus, tomato and walnuts. Then top with egg and season with pepper to taste, a dash of turmeric and olive oil.

Serve. Break egg yolk over top of quinoa and vegetables just before eating.

TIP Preparing quinoa in advance saves time on busy mornings. Just reheat in microwave before serving. Poached eggs may be stored in ice water overnight in fridge and reheated the next day by placing them in heated water (about 140 degrees) for 2 minutes.

SCIENCE & NUTRITION

Avocado + Tomato: The lipid content of avocado enhances absorption of the carotenoids found in tomato. Together, avocado and tomato deliver potent antioxidants as well as healthy fats that benefit skin by scavenging radicals and improving cellular function.

- *Unlu, N., et al. "Carotenoid absorption from salad and salsa by humans is enhanced by the addition of avocado or avocado oil," The Journal of Nutrition. 2005 Mar.; 135(3): 431-436.*

Romaine + Tomato + Quinoa: The antioxidant ferulic acid found in romaine and tomato can help stabilize vitamin E, of which quinoa is an excellent source. When coupled with ferulic acid, vitamin E's protective benefits against skin photoaging are 200% of those registered without concurrent consumption of ferulic acid.

- *Graf, E. "Antioxidant potential of ferulic acid," Free Radical Biology and Medicine. 1992 Oct.; 13(4): 435-448.*

- *Lin, F., et al. "Ferulic acid stabilizes a solution of vitamins C and E and doubles its photoprotection of skin," Journal of Investigative Dermatology. 2005; 125: 826-832.*

450 calories; 26g fat; 4g sat. fat; 215mg cholesterol; 80mg sodium; 630mg potassium; 43g carbohydrates; 9g fiber; 7g sugar; 16g protein. 2 servings.

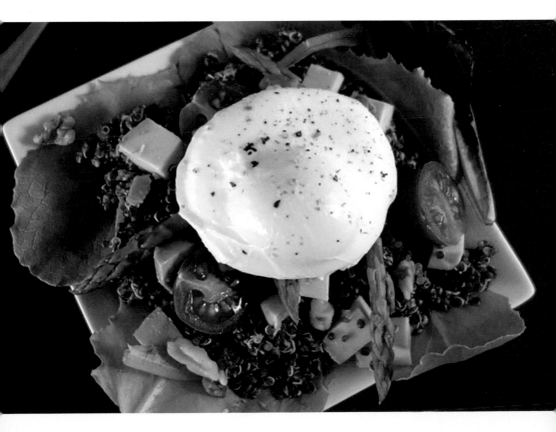

NO-MORE-DARK-SPOTS OATS

½ **cup gluten-free rolled oats, dry**

1 **tsp. unrefined coconut oil, melted**

2 **tsp. honey**

¼ **tsp. cinnamon**

½ **tsp. chia seeds**

¼ **cup blueberries**

2 **tbsp. pomegranate seeds**

5 **to 10 walnuts, roughly chopped**

Place dry oats in a small bowl. Do not cook.

Stir in coconut oil, honey, cinnamon, and chia seeds. Top with blueberries, pomegranate seeds, and walnuts. Serve.

SCIENCE & NUTRITION

Blueberries: Blueberries are a natural source of arbutin, a powerful skin lightener that is effective at reducing pigmentation inconsistencies in skin. Arbutin is similar in structure (and convertible to) hydroquinone, the active ingredient in popular skin-lightening creams.

- *Seo, D., et al. "Biotechnological production of arbutins (a- and B-arbutins), skin lightening agents, and their derivatives," Applied Microbiology and Biotechnology. 2012 Sep.; 95(6): 1417-1425.*

- *Jeon, J., et al. "Simultaneous determination of arbutin and its decomposed product hydroquinone in whitening creams using high-performance liquid chromatography with photodiode array detection: effect of temperature and pH on decomposition," International Journal of Cosmetic Science. 2015.*

Pomegranate Seeds: The ellagic acid found in pomegranate seeds has been found effective at reducing and treating UV-induced photodamage, thus helping resolve a main factor in skin aging and the production of dark spots in skin.

- *Hseu, Y., et al. "Ellagic acid protects human keratinocyte (HaCaT) cells against UVA-induced oxidative stress and apoptosis through the upregulation of the HO-1 and Nrf-2 antioxidant genes," Food and Chemical Toxicology. 2012 May; 50(5): 1245-1255.*

460 calories; 26g fat; 7g sat. fat; 0mg cholesterol; 10mg sodium; 210mg potassium; 52g carbohydrates; 9g fiber; 19g sugar; 11g protein. 1 serving.

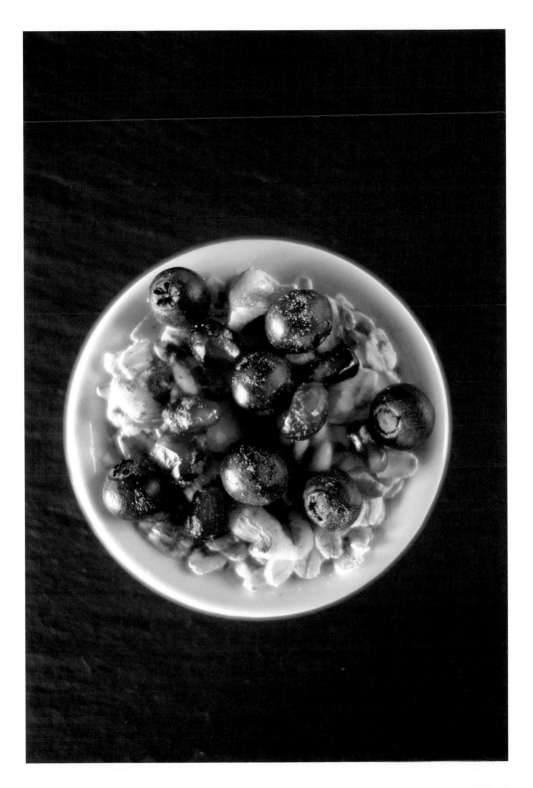

MAKE-YOUR-SKIN-GLOW SPINACH & EGGS

¼ cup dry wild rice, prepared according to package instructions

2 tsp. extra virgin olive oil + extra for seasoning

Heaping handful baby spinach leaves

¼ small heirloom tomato, diced

1 garlic clove, minced or crushed

Ground black pepper

2 tsp. white wine vinegar

1 tsp. sea salt + extra for seasoning

2 eggs, chilled

Prepare rice according to package instructions.

Heat small skillet over medium heat. Pour 1 tsp. olive oil into skillet and swirl to coat. Once oil is warm, add spinach, tomato, and garlic. Sauté until spinach is just wilted. Season with salt and pepper to taste. Set spinach mixture aside in small bowl.

Fill a large, deep non-stick skillet 1½ inches deep with water and heat over medium heat. Stir in vinegar and 1 tsp. salt. While water heats, crack each egg into a separate ramekin and set aside.

Once vinegar water reaches simmer, slowly lower ramekins into water, allowing eggs to enter water. Do not agitate the egg whites or they will feather. Turn off heat, cover and let eggs poach for 5 minutes. Do not disturb eggs while poaching. Meanwhile, line a plate with paper towels.

Remove eggs from water with a slotted spoon and place on paper towel lined plate to drain water.

Place cooked rice in a bowl. Top with spinach mixture and poached eggs. Drizzle with olive oil and season to taste with salt and pepper. Enjoy.

SCIENCE & NUTRITION

Tomato + Egg + Spinach: Carotenoids and phenolics, when consumed together, exhibit synergistic antioxidant effects, protecting the body and skin from oxidative damage. Tomato and eggs are both excellent sources of highly bioavailable carotenoids, and there is evidence that egg consumption enhances the body's absorption of plant-based carotenoid antioxidants. Since spinach is rich in phenolic antioxidants, consuming these foods all at once enhances their antioxidant benefits for skin.

- *Milde, J., et al. "Synergistic effects of phenolics and carotenoids on human low-density lipoprotein oxidation," Molecular Nutrition and Food Research. 2007 Aug.; 51(8): 956-961.*

- *Kim, J.E., et al. "Effects of egg consumption on carotenoid absorption from co-consumed, raw vegetables," The American Journal of Clinical Nutrition. 2015; ajcn111062.*

- *Pandjaitan, N., et al. "Antioxidant capacity and phenolic content of spinach as affected by genetics and maturation," Journal of Agricultural and Food Chemistry. 2005 Nov.; 53(22): 8618-8623.*

Tomato + Olive Oil: The antioxidant activity of lycopene from tomatoes is enhanced by about 20% when consumed with olive oil.

- *Lee, A., et al. "Consumption of tomato products with olive oil but not sunflower oil increases the antioxidant activity of plasma," Free Radical Biology and Medicine. 2000 Nov.; 29(10): 1051-1055.*

400 calories; 21g fat; 4g sat. fat; 430mg cholesterol; 540mg sodium; 620mg potassium; 37g carbohydrates; 5g fiber; 2g sugar; 20g protein. 1 serving.

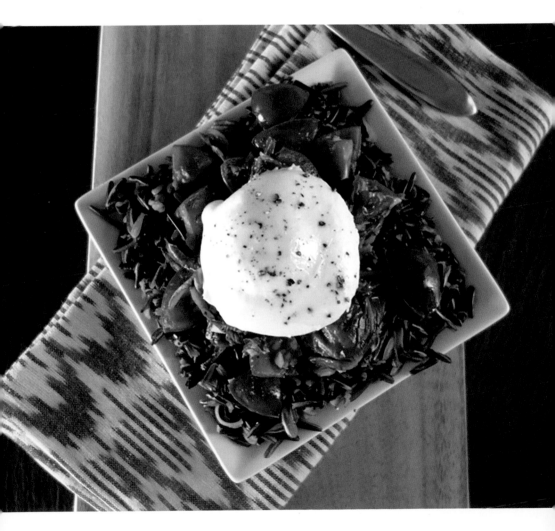

NATURAL SUNSCREEN GREEN EGGS & OMEGAS

1 avocado, sliced in half with pit and skin removed

2 tsp. white wine vinegar

1 tsp. salt + extra for seasoning

2 eggs, chilled

¼ cup mini heirloom tomatoes, halved

2-3 basil leaves, julienned

¼ lime

Ground black pepper, to taste

Sea salt

Fill a large, deep non-stick skillet 1½ inches deep with water and heat over medium heat. Stir in vinegar and 1 tsp. salt. While water heats, crack each egg into a separate ramekin and set aside.

Once vinegar water reaches simmer, slowly lower ramekins into water, allowing eggs to enter water. Do not agitate the egg whites or they will feather. Turn off heat, cover and let eggs poach for 5 minutes. Do not disturb eggs while poaching. Meanwhile, line a plate with paper towels. Slice, pit and peel avocado.

Remove eggs from water with a slotted spoon and place on paper towel lined plate to drain water.

Top each avocado half with a poached egg (place in hole where pit has been removed), tomatoes and basil. Season with salt and pepper, squeeze lime juice on top and drizzle with olive oil. Serve.

SCIENCE & NUTRITION

Avocado + Tomato: Using different chemical pathways, both avocado and tomato protect the skin from UV-related photoaging. The two foods complement one another to enhance skin's resilience to sun exposure and arrest skin photoaging.

- *Rosenblat, G., et al. "Polyhydroxylated fatty alcohols derived from avocado suppress inflammatory response and provide non-sunscreen protection against UV-induced damage in skin cells," Archives of Dermatological Research. 2011 May; 303(4): 239-246.*

- *Rizwan, M., et al. "Tomato paste rich in lycopene protects against cutaneous photodamage in humans in vivo: a randomized controlled trial," British Journal of Dermatology. 2011 Jan.; 164(1): 154-162.*

Basil: Along with its antioxidant and anti-inflammatory properties, basil has been shown to exhibit sunscreen activity (in topical applications), suggesting that consumption of basil can disrupt the chemical pathways leading to skin photodamage.

- *Balakrishnan, K.P., et al. "Botanicals as sunscreens: their role in the prevention of photoaging and skin cancer," International Journal of Research in Cosmetic Science. 2011; 1(1): 1-12.*

250 calories; 19g fat; 4g sat. fat; 215mg cholesterol; 190mg sodium; 710mg potassium; 14g carbohydrates; 8g fiber; 3g sugar; 9g protein. 2 servings.

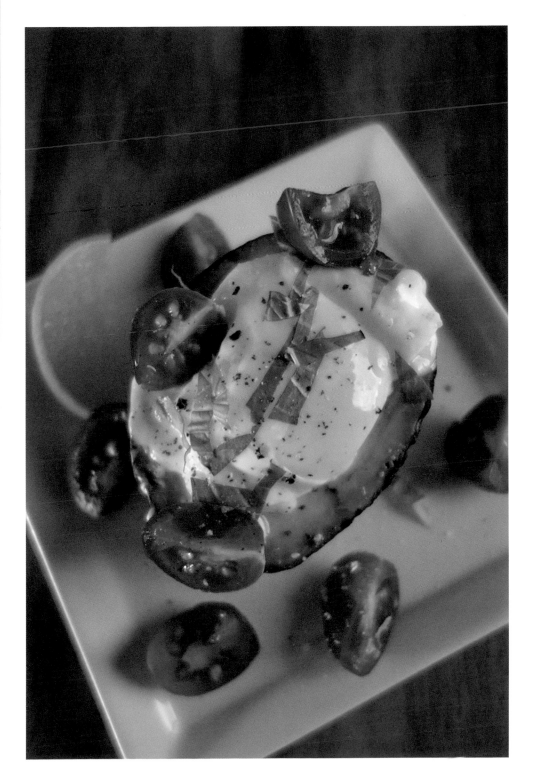

SKIN-PLUMPING BERRY SMOOTHIE

1 heaping cup frozen mixed berries, thawed at room temperature for 5 to 10 minutes

2 oz. fresh-squeezed orange juice

½ tbsp. chia seeds

1 tbsp. unrefined coconut oil, melted

1 ripe banana, including about 2 square inches of peel, washed and dried

Place all ingredients in a blender and blend until smooth, about 1 minute. Serve.

SCIENCE & NUTRITION

Chia Seeds: The ALA Omega-3 fatty acids in chia seeds provide beneficial fats for healthy, plump skin cells. ALA fatty acids, derived from plants, can be converted in the human body to EPA and DHA type Omega-3 fatty acids for use in the body's functions. It is recommended that both plant-based and ani-mal-based Omega-3 fatty acids be consumed in the diet for optimal health and skin outcomes.

- *Barcelo-Coblijn, G., et al. "Alpha-linolenic acid and its conversion to longer chain n-3 fatty acids: benefits for human health and a role in maintaining tissue n-3 fatty acid levels," Progress in Lipid Research. 2009 Nov.; 48(6): 355-374.*

Banana Peel: The antifungal and antibiotic structures found within banana peels benefit skin health by reducing inflammation and skin irritation from environ-mental factors and disease agents.

- *Sampath Kumar, K.P., et al. "Traditional and medicinal uses of banana," Journal of Pharmacognosy and Phytochemistry. 2012; 1(3): 51-63.*

180 calories; 8g fat; 6g sat. fat; 0mg cholesterol; 10mg sodium; 370mg potassium; 26g carbohydrates; 5g fiber; 16g sugar; 2g protein. 2 servings.

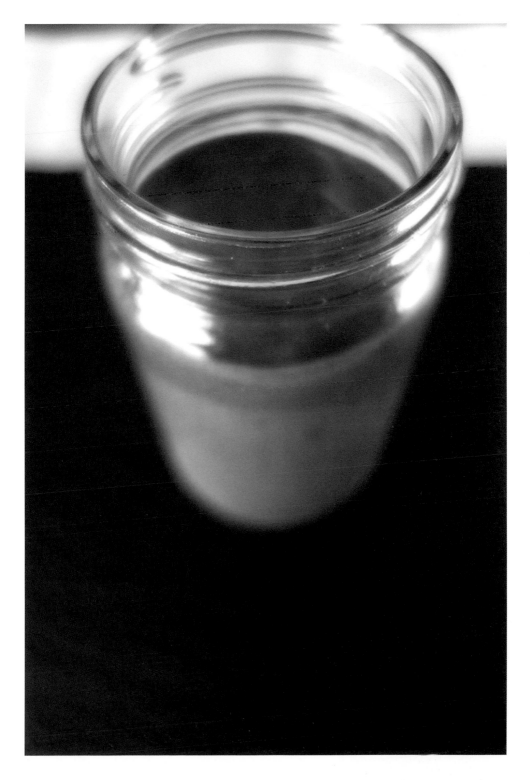

BLEMISH CONTROL FRUIT TEA CUP

½ **apple, diced**

12 red grapes, halved

1 serving peppermint tea or ginger pear tea, brewed and chilled

2 to 3 mint leaves, chopped

Place fruit in a glass serving dish or cup. Pour tea over fruit until just covered. Sprinkle mint leaves on top and serve with a spoon.

SCIENCE & NUTRITION

Red Grapes: The antioxidant resveratrol is found in red grapes, but is otherwise unlikely to be found in the diet. Resveratrol protects skin from ultraviolet radiation and other damage, helping skin remain healthy and youthful despite UV exposure.

- *Ndiaye, M., et al. "The grape antioxidant resveratrol for skin disorders: promise, prospects, and challenges," Archives of Biochemistry and Biophysics. 2011 Apr.; 508(2): 164-170.*

Mint: The oil from mint has anti-inflammatory, antiviral and antibacterial properties that help keep infections at bay, allowing skin to maintain a healthy and youthful appearance.

- *Chawla, S., et al. "Overview of mint (mentha l.) as a promising health-promoting herb," International Journal of Pharmaceutical Research and Development. 2013 Aug.; 5(6): 73-80.*

40 calories; 0g fat; 0g sat. fat; 0mg cholesterol; 0mg sodium; 80mg potassium; 9g carbohydrates; 1g fiber; 7g sugar; 0g protein. 2 servings.

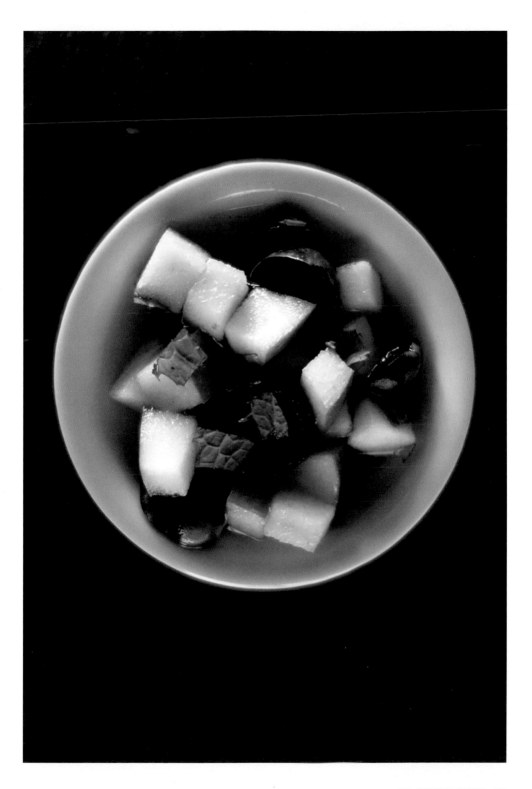

COLLAGEN-BOOSTING STRAWBERRY-MELON REFRESH

1 heaping cup frozen strawberries, thawed

Allow strawberries to thaw at room temperature for 20 to 30 minutes.

1 heaping cup fresh seedless watermelon, cubed and refrigerated

Combine strawberries, watermelon cubes, lime juice, and lime zest in a blender. Blend until smooth. Serve immediately.

Juice from 1 lime

¼ tsp. lime zest

SCIENCE & NUTRITION

Strawberry: Strawberries exhibit strong inhibition activity against advanced glycation end product formation. Advanced glycation end products cause oxidative stress in the body linked with aging, including the degradation of skin collagen. By countering the formation of advanced glycation end products, strawberries help maintain and promote young-looking skin.

- *Parengkuan, L., et al. "Anti-glycation activity of various fruits," Anti-Aging Medicine. 2013; 10(4): 70-76.*

Lime Peel + Lime Juice: The peel of citrus fruits, like lime, contain powerful phenolics, flavonoids and carotenoids that provide antioxidant benefits. Coupled with the antioxidant punch of juice of lime, the antioxidants in peel and juice can behave synergistically to provide significant scavenging of free radicals and thus forestall skin aging.

- *Guimaraes, R., et al. "Targeting excessive free radicals with peels and juices of citrus fruits: grapefruit, lemon, lime and orange," Food and Chemical Toxicology. 2010 Jan.; 48(1): 99-106.*

140 calories; 0g fat; 0g sat. fat; 0mg cholesterol; 0mg sodium; 440mg potassium; 35g carbohydrates; 5g fiber; 24g sugar; 2g protein. 1 serving.

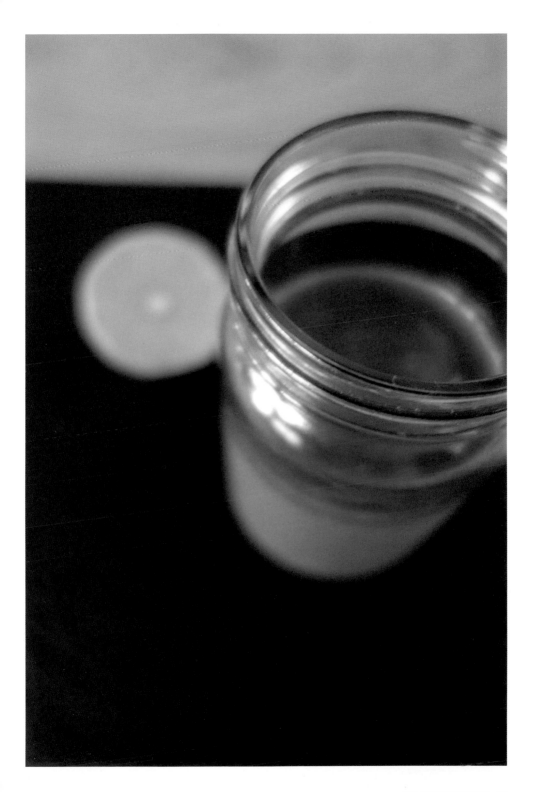

HEALTHY SKIN PISTACHIO-MELON-CHERRY PANACHE

¼ large watermelon, chilled and sliced into 1-inch cubes

12 cherries, pits and stems removed

¼ cup unsalted pistachio nutmeats

Juice from ¼ lime + ¼ tsp. lime zest

Place all ingredients except lime juice and zest into serving bowls. Squeeze lime juice over top, sprinkle with lime zest, and serve.

SCIENCE & NUTRITION

Watermelon + Pistachios: Using two different biochemical pathways, both watermelon and pistachios improve circulatory function. The two ingredients combined offer a super shot of circulatory boost to move nutrients to cells and clear waste. The fats and protein in pistachios blunt the impact of watermelon's sugar on the body's systems, thereby strengthening the foods' synergistic interplay.

- *Collins, J., et al. "Watermelon consumption increases plasma arginine concentration in adults," Nutrition. 2007 Mar.; 23(3): 261-266.*

- *Sheridan, M., et al. "Pistachio nut consumption and serum lipid levels," Journal of the American College of Nutrition. 2007; 26(2): 141-148.*

Cherries: Anthocyanins in cherries have been shown to significantly reduce systemic and local inflammation and can thus enhance skin appearance by calming skin cells and by promoting cellular metabolic efficiency.

- *Jacob, R., et al. "Consumption of cherries lowers plasma urate in healthy women," The Journal of Nutrition. 2003 Jun.; 133(6): 1826-1829.*

- *Kelley, D., et al. "Consumption of bing sweet cherries lowers circulating concentrations of inflammation markers in healthy men and women," The Journal of Nutrition. 2006 Apr.; 136(4): 981-986.*

180 calories; 8g fat; 1g sat. fat; 0mg cholesterol; 10mg sodium; 490mg potassium; 28g carbohydrates; 3g fiber; 18g sugar; 5g protein. 2 servings.

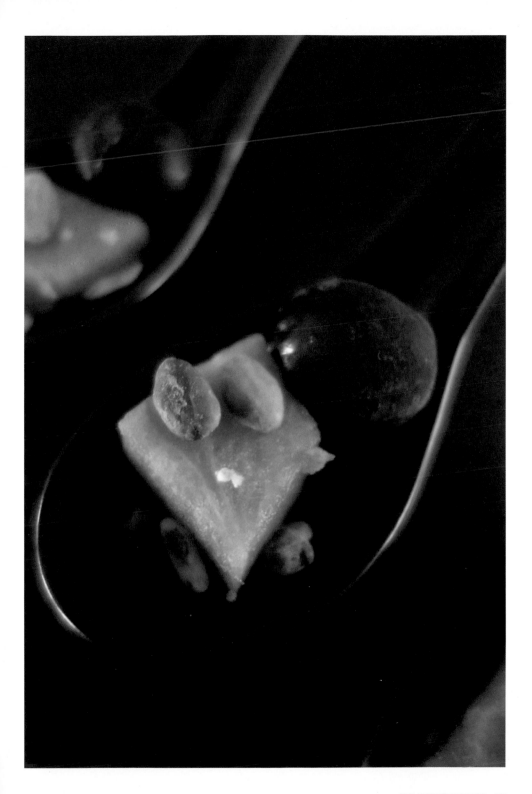

THE **YOUNG SKIN** DIET

LUNCHES

STRESS-FIGHTING SALMON CAKES

6 oz. canned wild salmon, including juices

¼ cup + 2 tsp. gluten-free oat flour (or more, as needed to form patties)

1 egg, lightly beaten

2 tsp. Trader Joe's Chili Pepper Sauce (or another sodium-free hot sauce)

¼ tsp. ground black pepper

Extra virgin olive oil

½ lemon

Mix ingredients together in a medium bowl. Form 4 salmon patties and then squeeze lemon juice onto patties.

Heat non-stick skillet over medium to medium-high heat. Add a just enough olive oil to lightly coat the bottom of the skillet. Swirl to coat evenly.

Heat patties in skillet for 3 to 4 minutes per side. Serve.

SCIENCE & NUTRITION

Chili Pepper Sauce: The capsaicin found in hot peppers provides potent antioxidant effects that offer protection against age-related disease and age-related changes in skin appearance.

- *Luqman, S. et al. "Protection of lipid peroxidation and carbonyl formation in proteins by capsaicin in human erythrocytes subjected to oxidative stress," Phytotherapy Research. 2006 Apr.; 20(4): 303-306.*

Salmon + Lemon: The EPA and DHA long-chain Omega-3 fatty acids from salmon ameliorate chronic health problems associated with inflammation. These inflammation-related problems affect the body's entire ecosystem, including the gut, joints, brain, cardiovascular complex and skin. Improving function across the entire system promotes healthy and youthful skin by ensuring the body's resources are appropriately directed to the skin for healing and repair. Citrus juices like lemon reduce advanced glycation end product formation in salmon as it cooks.

- *Wall, R., et al. "Fatty acids from fish: the anti-inflammatory potential of long-chain omega-3 fatty acids," Nutrition Reviews. 2010; 68(5): 280-289.*

- *Kris-Etherton, P., et al. "Fish consumption, fish oil, omega-3 fatty acids, and cardiovascular disease," Circulation. 2002; 106: 2747-2757.*

- *Uribarri, J., et al. "Advanced glycation end products in foods and a practical guide to their reduction in the diet," Journal of the American Dietetic Association. 2010 Jun.; 110(6): 911-916.*

120 calories; 5g fat; 1g sat. fat; 77mg cholesterol; 50mg sodium; 180mg potassium; 7g carbohydrates; 1g fiber; 0g sugar; 11g protein. 4 servings.

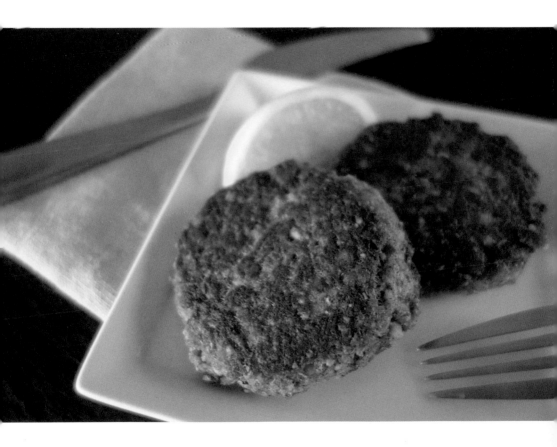

REPAIR-YOUR-SKIN THAI QUINOA & KALE SALAD

1 cup dry red or white quinoa

14 oz. low fat coconut milk

2 tbsp. red curry paste

½ tbsp. palm sugar

10 oz. chopped kale, stems removed

1 cup shredded cabbage

1 cup shredded carrots

½ red bell pepper, diced and sautéed

½ yellow onion, diced and sautéed

¼ cup roasted, unsalted cashews

1 lime, quartered

Sea salt

Prepare quinoa according to package instructions, using coconut milk in place of water. While quinoa heats, stir in curry paste and palm sugar. Continue cooking until liquid is absorbed.

Fill a large pot with water, add a dash of salt and bring to a boil.

When water reaches boil, insert kale and boil for 3 to 4 minutes. Remove kale with tongs, place in a colander and rinse with cold water. Boil cabbage and carrots in water for 90 seconds. Place carrots and cabbage in colander with kale and rinse with cold water.

Pat vegetables dry and place them in a large mixing bowl. Add quinoa mixture, red pepper, onion and cashews. Toss ingredients and squeeze lime over salad and sprinkle with salt to taste.

TIP For extra skin benefits and less work in the kitchen, serve kale, shredded cabbage, and carrots raw.

SCIENCE & NUTRITION

Kale + Lime: The nutrient density of kale is exceptionally high, and the vitamin C from lime helps the body absorb those nutrients, particularly the iron. Iron helps keep the circulatory system efficient and assists in cellular repair, reducing the incidence of damaged cells in the skin, the presence of which can be responsible for aged, rough, wrinkled and sagging skin.

- *Hallberg, L., et al. "The role of vitamin C in iron absorption," International Journal of Vitamin and Nutrition Research. 1989; 30: 103-108.*

Cashews: Healthy fats and minerals are found in abundance in cashews, making them an excellent resource for skin repair and health.

- *Ros, E., et al. "Fatty acid composition of nuts – implications for cardiovascular health," British Journal of Nutrition. 2006 Nov.; 96 (Supp. 2): S29-S35.*
- *Brufau, G., et al. "Nuts: source of energy and macronutrients," British Journal of Nutrition. 2006 Nov.; 96(Supp. 2): S22-S28.*

Quinoa: Endowed with lysine, quinoa presents a complete protein from its amino acid profile, providing the essential building blocks for new skin cells, new collagen and healthy facial muscles, all of which contribute to young-looking skin.

- *Abugoch, J. "Quinoa (chenopodium quinoa willd.): composition, chemistry, nutritional, and functional properties," Advances in Food and Nutrition Research. 2009; 58: 1-31.*

- *Vega-Galvez, A., et al. "Nutrition facts and functional potential of quinoa (chenopodium quinoa willd.), an ancient Andean grain: a review," Journal of the Science of Food Agriculture. 2010 Dec.; 90(15): 2541-2547.*

350 calories; 11g fat; 4g sat. fat; 0mg cholesterol; 260mg sodium; 570mg potassium; 55g carbohydrates; 9g fiber; 12g sugar; 12g protein. 4 servings.

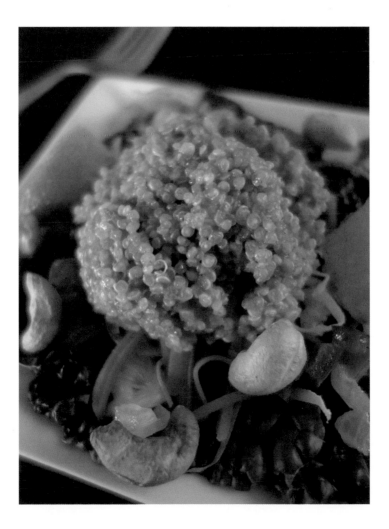

REJUVENATING MYKONOS MEDITERRANEAN SALAD

SALAD
1 dozen cherry tomatoes, halved

1 cucumber, chopped into ¼ inch rounds

½ cup kalamata olives

¼ red onion, thinly sliced

2 anchovy fillets in extra virgin olive oil, chopped into fine pieces

DRESSING
¼ cup extra virgin olive oil

1 tbsp. lemon juice

1 garlic clove, minced

1 tsp. Dijon mustard

Sea salt (to taste)

Place all dressing ingredients in a resealable container and shake vigorously.

Place all salad ingredients in a large bowl. Pour dressing over salad and toss to coat. Serve.

SCIENCE & NUTRITION

Anchovies in Extra Virgin Olive Oil: The beneficial fatty acid content and composition of anchovies (and other fatty fish) stored in extra virgin olive oil remains highest relative to other storing liquids like seed oils. Selecting anchovies stored in extra virgin olive oil ensures the highest efficacy of Omega-3 fatty acids for smooth and strong skin.

- *Caponio, F. et al. "Fatty acid composition and degradation level of the oils used in canned fish as a function of the different types of fish," Journal of Food Composition and Analysis. 2011 Dec.; 24(8): 1117-1122.*

Kalamata Olives: Phenolic compounds in kalamata olives are powerful anti-inflammatories, which enable efficient cellular function. Unlike some olives, kalamata olives tend not to be chemically treated in preparation for human consumption, so their phenols are not disrupted by chemical processing that can interfere with antioxidant and anti-inflammatory benefits.

- *Dimitrios, B. "Sources of natural phenolic antioxidants," Trends in Food Science & Technology. 2006 Sep.; 17(9): 505-512.*

Cucumber + Anchovies: Cucumber provides water and potassium, which help balance the sodium from salts found in anchovies to enable efficient cellular function. Good cellular function results in optimal cell volume and thus contributes to smooth and healthy skin.

- *Tanase, C., et al. "Sodium and potassium in composite food samples from the Canadian total diet study," Journal of Food Composition and Analysis. 2011 Mar.; 24(2): 237-243.*

350 calories; 33g fat; 4g sat. fat; 4mg cholesterol; 460mg sodium; 470mg potassium; 14g carbohydrates; 2g fiber; 7g sugar; 3g protein. 2 servings.

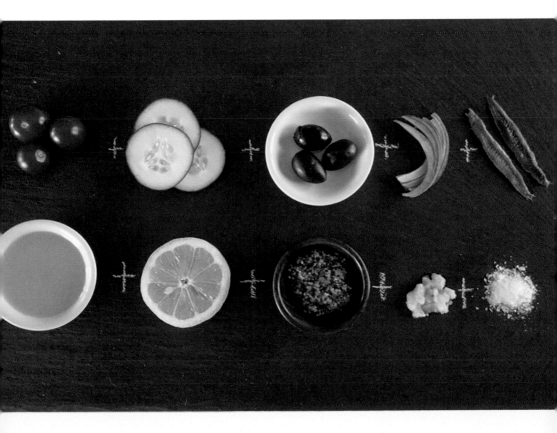

YOUNG SKIN CURRY SOUP

2 tsp. unrefined coconut oil

½ cup red onion, chopped

2 cups carrots, peeled and sliced into ¼-inch rounds

2 cups sweet potatoes, cut into ½-inch cubes with skin left on

½ tbsp. ginger, peeled and grated

1 tsp. cumin

½ tsp. coriander

½ tsp. allspice

¼ tsp. salt

¼ tsp. cinnamon

3 cups low-sodium vegetable broth

1 cup low fat coconut milk

Heat coconut oil in a large stockpot over medium to medium-high heat. Add onion and sauté until translucent, about 2 minutes. Add remaining vegetables, ginger and spices. Sauté for 2 more minutes.

Add vegetable stock and bring to a boil. Reduce heat to simmer, cover and cook until vegetables are tender, about 35 to 45 minutes. Stir in coconut milk.

Transfer pot contents in 2 to 3 batches to a food processor. Pulse until smooth. Serve immediately.

SCIENCE & NUTRITION

Red Onion: With stronger free radical scavenging activity than yellow onion or even garlic, red onion provides significant antioxidant action in the body to promote healthy, youthful skin.

- *Nuutila, A.M., et al. "Comparison of antioxidant activities of onion and garlic extracts by inhibition of lipid peroxidation and radical scavenging activity," Food Chemistry. 2003 Jun.; 81(4): 485-493.*

- *Prakash, D. "Antioxidant and free radical scavenging activities of phenols from onion (allium cepa)," Food Chemistry. 2007; 102(4): 1389-1393.*

Ginger + Cumin + Coriander + Allspice + Cinnamon: Spices, including those used here, provide concentrated and varied antioxidants, which remove the precursors of oxidative damage and skin aging from the body. Antioxidant activity of these spices is enhanced by cooking them in a soup preparation involving long heating times.

- *Yanishlieva, N., et al. "Natural antioxidants from herbs and spices," European Journal of Lipid Science and Technology. 2006 Sep.; 108(9): 776-793.*

- *Khatum, M., et al. "Effect of thermal treatment on radical-scavenging activity of some spices," Food Science and Technology Research. 2006; 12(3): 178-185.*

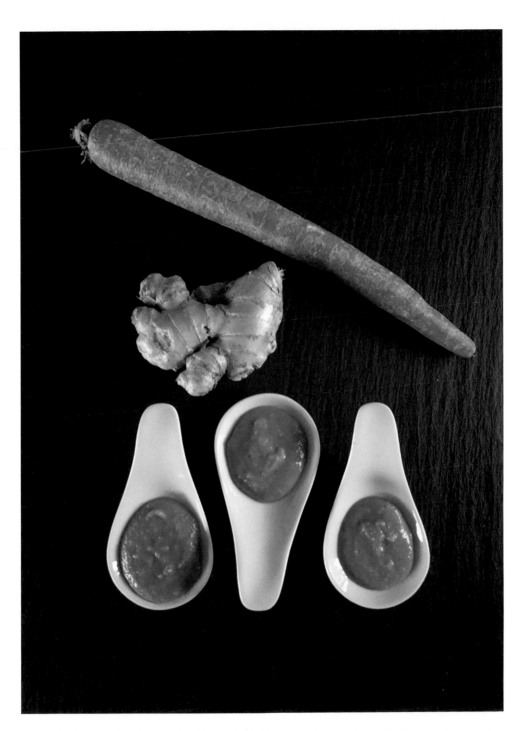

160 calories; 5g fat; 4g sat. fat; 0mg cholesterol; 310mg sodium; 450mg potassium; 27g carbohydrates; 6g fiber; 10g sugar; 3g protein. 4 servings.

SMOOTH SKIN ZUCCHINI WITH CHICKEN

6 zucchini, sliced ¼-inch thick lengthwise

Extra virgin olive oil

1 lb. chicken thighs

4 lemon wedges

2 garlic cloves, crushed

6 sprigs rosemary

½ tsp. sea salt + extra for seasoning

½ tsp. ground black pepper + extra for seasoning

1 cup white wine

Preheat oven to 450 degrees. Line a baking sheet with foil.

Toss zucchini with olive oil to lightly coat outsides. Season to taste with salt and pepper. Place on foiled-lined baking sheet. Bake in oven for 45 minutes, flipping zucchini halfway through baking time. Zucchini is ready when it has reduced in size and lost its firmness.

While zucchini bakes, place chicken in a single layer in a 2 to 4 quart pot. Scatter lemon, garlic, rosemary, salt and pepper on top. Pour wine over chicken. Pour cold water over chicken until covered by about an inch of liquid.

Bring liquid to a boil. Reduce heat to simmer, cover and cook until the center of meat registers 180 degrees, about 15 to 20 minutes.

Remove chicken from pot and let rest on cutting board for 2 to 3 minutes. Discard lemon wedges and rosemary sprigs. Serve chicken in bowls, ladling broth over meat until covered. Season with additional black pepper if desired. Serve roasted zucchini separately as a side.

SCIENCE & NUTRITION

Zucchini: Manganese found in zucchini is necessary for the body's use of choline. Choline, which is found in chicken and used in the formation of collagen, has been shown to enhance skin smoothness.

- Barel, A., et al. "Effect of oral intake of choline-stabilized orthosilicic acid on skin, nails and hair in women with photodamaged skin," Archives of Dermatologic Research. 2005 Oct.; 297(4): 147-153.

- Watts, D. "The nutritional relationships of manganese," Journal of Orthomolecular Medicine. 1990; 5(4): 219-222.

Chicken: Poultry, including chicken, is one of the best sources of carnosine and dipeptides used in the production of beta-alanine. Carnosine has been shown to reduce protein cross-linking in the skin and to thus ward off wrinkles and other signs of aging.

- Hipkiss, A.R. "Carnosine, a protective ,anti-ageing peptide?" Cell Biology. 1998 Aug.; 30(8): 863-868.

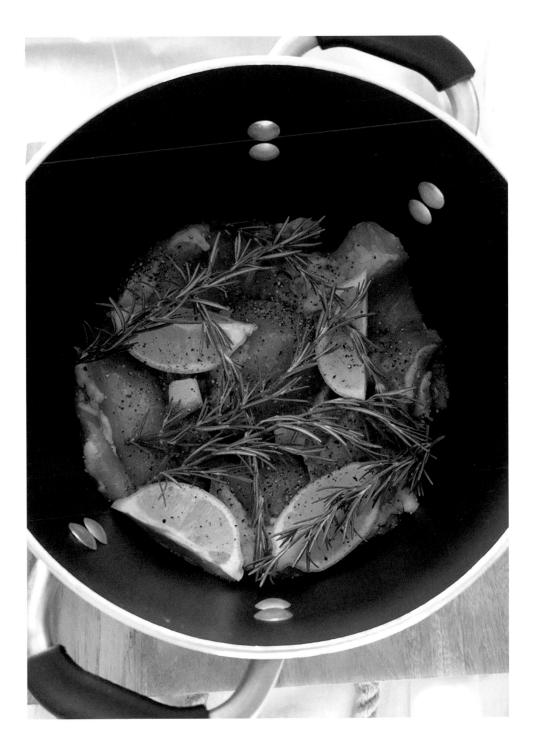

260 calories; 5g fat; 0g sat. fat; 96mg cholesterol; 180mg sodium; 1,120mg potassium; 18g carbohydrates; 5g fiber; 6g sugar; 40g protein. 4 servings.

SKIN-HEALING KALE SALAD WITH LEMON VINAIGRETTE

SALAD

1 head of garlic, top ¼-inch of cloves chopped off with outer skin removed

½ tsp. extra virgin olive oil

10 oz. chopped kale, stems removed

1 cup cabbage, shredded

2 handfuls walnuts

DRESSING

¼ cup extra virgin olive oil

¼ cup fresh-squeezed lemon juice

3 garlic cloves, minced

1 tsp. dried oregano

1 tsp. honey

½ tsp. ground black pepper

½ tsp. thyme

½ tsp. rosemary

⅛ tsp. salt

Preheat oven to 400 degrees.

Place garlic head on a sheet of foil and drizzle ½ tsp. olive oil on cut end of head. Rub olive oil over the cloves to ensure it coats the tops.

Wrap foil entirely around garlic, place foil-wrapped head on baking sheet, and bake until cloves are soft, about 30 to 35 minutes. Cloves are ready when they can be removed from their skin with a butter knife.

Vigorously mix dressing ingredients together in a small bowl or shake tightly in a sealed glass jar.

Place kale and cabbage in a large bowl and toss with dressing until leaves are thoroughly coated.

Dish into serving bowls. Top with walnuts and roasted garlic cloves. Serve.

SCIENCE & NUTRITION

Kale: Consumption of kale in raw form maximizes its available nutrients, poly-phenolic antioxidants and vitamin C, all of which contribute to smooth and healthy skin.

- *Sikora, E., et al. "Composition and antioxidant activity of kale (brassica oleracea l. var. acephala) raw and cooked," ACTA Scientarium Polonorum Technologia Alimentaria 2012; 11(3): 239-248.*

Cabbage: Cabbage contains the isoflavonoid equol, which exhibits strong anti-oxidant activity in the skin and which can improve collagen and elastin levels, as well as promote wound healing.

- *Lephart, E. "Human skin gene expression, attributes of botanicals: angelica sinensis, a soy extract, equol and its isomers and resveratrol," Gene Technology. 2015 Apr.; 4(2): 119-127.*

Olive Oil + Garlic: Both olive oil and garlic feature prominently in the traditional Mediterranean diet, which has been shown to promote antioxidant capacity in the blood and to reduce body weight and age-related health disorders, includ-ing those manifesting in the skin.

- *Razquin, C., et al. "A 3 years follow-up of a Mediterranean diet rich in virgin olive oil is associated with high plasma antioxidant capacity and reduced body weight gain," European Journal of Clinical Nutrition. 2009; 63: 1387-1393.*

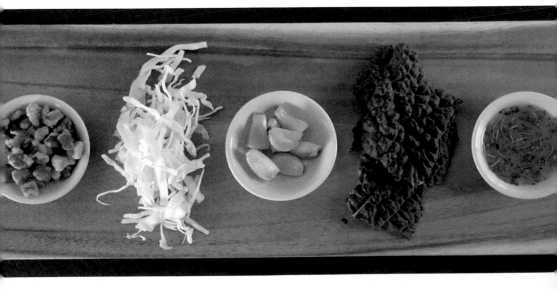

280 calories; 25g fat; 3g sat. fat; 0mg cholesterol; 100mg sodium; 430mg potassium; 17g carbohydrates; 3g fiber; 3g sugar; 6g protein. 4 servings.

THE **YOUNG SKIN** DIET

AFTERNOON SNACKS

COLLAGEN-BUILDING POMME SNACK

1 ripe Fuji, Red Delicious or Gala apple

1 tsp. unrefined coconut oil

Quatre épices spice mix (¼ tsp. allspice, ¼ tsp. nutmeg, ¼ tsp. cinnamon, and dash of cloves)

Slice apple into wedges, removing core.

Spread coconut oil atop apple slices and sprinkle with quatre épices mix. Serve.

SCIENCE & NUTRITION

Apple: The skin of apples contains vitamins that both help clear acne and build collagen and healthy, mature skin cells. Apples' phytochemicals help ward off oxidative damage and cancer activity. Among apple varieties, Fuji, Red Delicious and Gala (in that order) contain the highest concentrations of phenolics and flavonoids – up to twice as much as other apple varieties like Empire and Cortland.

- *Boyer, J., et al. "Apple phytochemicals and their health benefits," Nutrition Journal. 2004; 3: 5-21.*

Allspice + Nutmeg + Cinnamon + Cloves: These spices, cloves in particular, have highly concentrated levels of antioxidants that scavenge radicals from the body responsible for aging.

- *Yanishlieva, N., et al. "Natural antioxidants from herbs and spices," European Journal of Lipid Science and Technology. 2006 Sep.; 108(9): 776-793.*
- *Shan, B., et al. "Antioxidant capacity of 26 spice extracts and characterization of their phenolic constituents," Journal of Agricultural and Food Chemistry. 2005 Sep.; 53(20): 7749-7759.*

140 calories; 5g fat; 4g sat. fat; 0mg cholesterol; 2mg sodium; 200mg potassium; 25g carbohydrates; 4g fiber; 19g sugar; 0g protein. 1 serving.

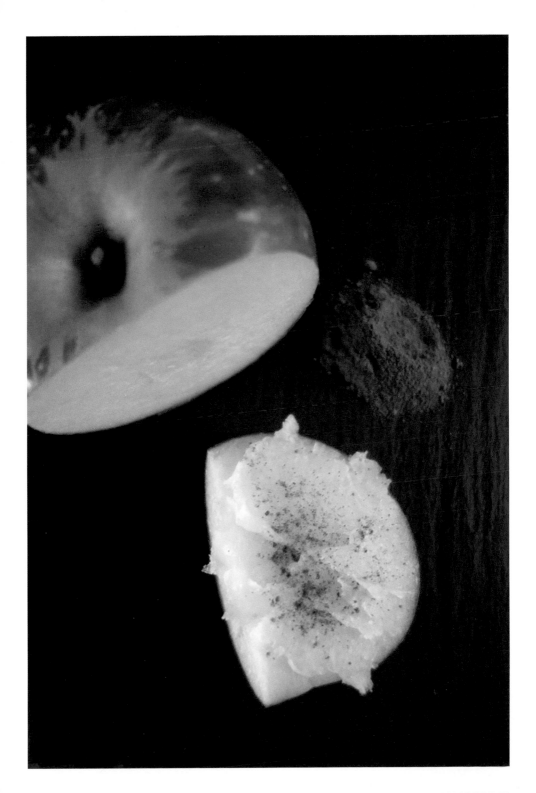

STRONG SKIN SPINACH AND CHICKPEAS

4 tbsp. extra virgin olive oil

1 yellow onion, thinly sliced

6 garlic cloves, minced

1 small, ripe tomato, diced

2 tsp. smoked paprika

1 tsp. cumin

¼ tsp. sea salt

15 oz. canned chickpeas, drained and rinsed

10 oz. baby spinach

Heat olive oil in a large, deep non-stick skillet over medium to medium-high heat. Add onion and garlic and sauté until onion is soft, about 3 minutes.

Add tomato, paprika, cumin, salt and chickpeas. Continue to cook over medium to medium-high heat, stirring frequently, until tomato begins to fall apart and chickpeas are heated through, about 5 minutes.

Stir in spinach and cook until spinach leaves are just wilted. Remove from heat and scoop mixture, including juices, into bowls and serve.

SCIENCE & NUTRITION

Chickpeas: Hyaluronic acid keeps the collagen matrix of the skin healthy. Chickpeas are a good source of hyaluronic acid, as well as silica, both of which are used to manufacture new collagen and to keep existing collagen and other connective tissues in the skin and body strong. Silica also is associated with efficient calcium usage, helping keep calcification in the bones and out of the skin.

- *Chen, W., et al. "Functions of hyaluronan in wound repair," Wound Repair and Regeneration. 1999 Mar.-Apr.; 7(2): 79-89.*
- *Jugdaohsing, R. "Silicon and bone health," Journal of Nutrition, Health & Aging. 2007 Mar.; 11(2): 99-110.*

Garlic: Allicin, a chemical in garlic, exhibits strong antimicrobial effects, beneficial for cellular health and repair. To unleash allicin, it is necessary to "damage" the garlic clove by mincing, dicing, etc. before consuming, as in this recipe.

- *Ankri, S., et al. "Antimicrobial properties of allicin from garlic," Microbes and Infection. 1999 Feb.; 1(2): 125-129.*

190 calories; 11g fat; 1g sat. fat; 0mg cholesterol; 340mg sodium; 440mg potassium; 17g carbohydrates; 6g fiber; 2g sugar; 6g protein. 6 servings.

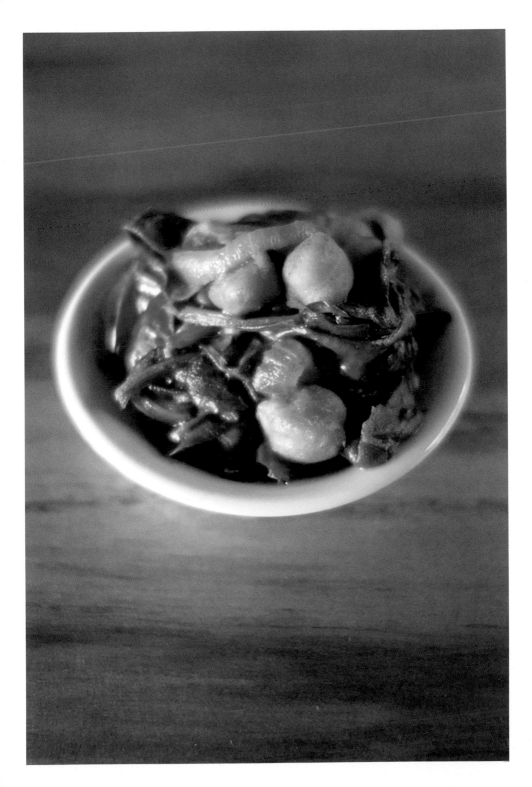

REVITALIZING GOJI GREATNESS

1 tbsp. flax meal

3 tbsp. water

3 tbsp. unrefined coconut oil, melted + ½ tsp.

2 tbsp. honey

½ tbsp. chia seeds

¾ tsp. cinnamon

¼ tsp. salt

¼ cup unsalted cashews, roughly chopped

¼ cup cashew butter

¾ cup gluten-free rolled oats

¼ cup goji berries

Preheat oven to 350 degrees and lightly coat a cookie sheet with ½ tsp. coconut oil.

Soak flax meal in water for 5 minutes.

In a medium bowl, combine flax meal mixture, coconut oil, honey, chia seeds, cinnamon, and salt. Stir in chopped cashews and cashew butter. Gradually stir in rolled oats and goji berries.

Pour mixture onto cookie sheet, forming a flat, roughly 4-inch-by-8-inch block. Bake until golden brown on edges, about 10 minutes.

Remove from oven and allow to cool completely. Slice into 8 square pieces and serve. Store remaining bars in an air-tight container in a cool, dry space.

TIP I recommend preparing this dish on the weekend to eat throughout the week. For homemade cashew butter, combine 1 cup of cashews with 1 to 2 tbsp. melted coconut oil. Process in food processor or blender on high speed until smooth.

SCIENCE & NUTRITION

Goji Berries: Goji berries have been shown to promote the release of progenitor cells in the body. Progenitor cells are believed to have a significant role in maintaining the health and vitality of many of the body's systems, including adult skin, thereby slowing various age-related processes in the skin such as dark spot formation, improving skin healing and contributing to youthful appearance.

- *Blanpain, C. and E. Fuchs. "Epidermal stem cells of the skin," Annual Review of Cell and Developmental Biology. 2006; 22: 339-373.*

- *Mikirova, N., et al. "Circulating endothelial progenitor cells: a new approach to anti-aging medicine?" Journal of Translational Medicine. 2009 Dec.; 7: 106-117.*

Cashews: Roasted cashews contain higher levels of antioxidant flavonoids than un-roasted cashews. The antioxidant profile of cashews is very strong and has been associated with myriad health benefits, including reduction in the loss of skin youthfulness.

- *Chandrasekara, N., et al. "Effect of roasting on phenolic content and antioxidant activities of whole cashew nuts, kernels, and testa," Journal of Agricultural and Food Chemistry. 2011; 59(9): 5006-5014.*

- *Suo, M., et al. "Phenolic lipid ingredients from cashew nuts," Journal of Natural Medicines. 2012 Jan.; 66(1): 133-139.*

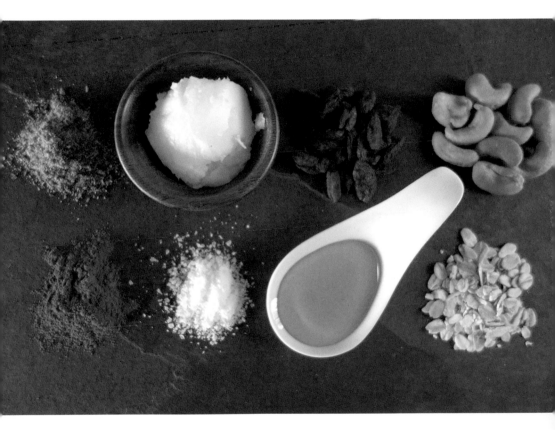

180 calories; 12g fat; 6g sat. fat; 0mg cholesterol; 70mg sodium; 60mg potassium; 16g carbohydrates; 2g fiber; 7g sugar; 4g protein. 8 servings.

RADIANT SKIN RED FRUIT MEDLEY

½ **Fuji, Red Delicious or Gala apple, chopped**

5 to 10 red grapes, halved

5 strawberries, halved

1 tbsp. chia seeds

Combine fruit ingredients in bowl.

Sprinkle with chia seeds. Serve.

SCIENCE & NUTRITION

Apples + Red Grapes + Strawberries: Apples, red grapes and strawberries are among the best sources of phenolic phytochemicals with antioxidant properties. The antioxidants present in these fruits work additively and synergistically when the foods are consumed together, providing significant radical scavenging and health protection benefits that, among other things, promote skin youthfulness by attenuating aging-related processes at a cellular level.

- Liu, R. "Potential synergy of phytochemicals in cancer prevention: mechanism of action," The Journal of Nutrition. 2004 Dec.; 134(12): 3479S-3485S.

- Liu, R. "Health benefits of fruit and vegetables are from additive and synergistic combinations of phytochemicals," The American Journal of Clinical Nutrition. 2003 Sep.; 78(3): 517S-520S.

150 calories; 5g fat; 1g sat. fat; 0mg cholesterol; 50mg sodium; 190mg potassium; 19g carbohydrates; 9g fiber; 14g sugar; 3g protein. 1 serving.

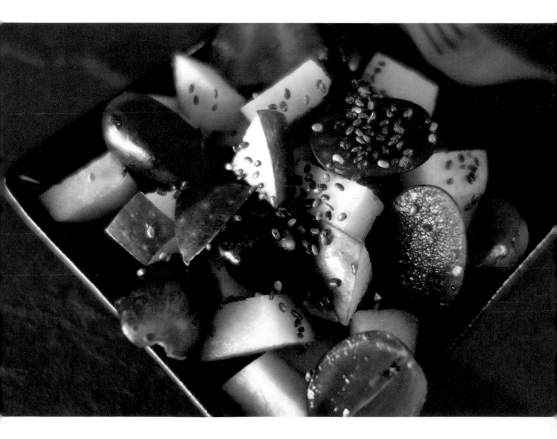

HYDRATING CUCUMBER & WATERMELON COOLDOWN

¼ **cucumber, diced**

1 cup watermelon, cubed

2 tsp. balsamic vinegar

2 to 3 mint leaves, chopped

¼ **tsp. ground black pepper**

Mix cucumber and watermelon in a bowl.

Drizzle with balsamic vinegar and sprinkle with mint leaves and black pepper. Serve.

SCIENCE & NUTRITION

Watermelon + Cucumber: Both watermelon and cucumber are excellent sources of hydration, which is necessary for cellular volume, skin moisture and clearance of waste from the body, all of which contributes to healthy and youthful skin. The balance of potassium and sodium electrolytes in watermelon and cucumber is also beneficial for hydration and mineral retention in the body, which keeps skin cells healthy.

- *He, F., et al. "Beneficial effects of potassium on human health," Physiologia Plantarum. 2008 Aug.; 133(4): 725-735.*

Cucumber: A source of bioaccessible silica, cucumber strengthens connective tissues, including the collagen matrix in the skin, which is comprised largely of silica.

- *Rani, B., et al. "Invigorating efficacy of cucumis sativas for healthcare & radiance," International Journal of Chemistry and Pharmaceutical Sciences. 2014; 2(3): 737-744.*

60 calories; 0g fat; 0g sat. fat; 0mg cholesterol; 0mg sodium; 280mg potassium; 15g carbohydrates; 1g fiber; 10g sugar; 1g protein. 1 serving.

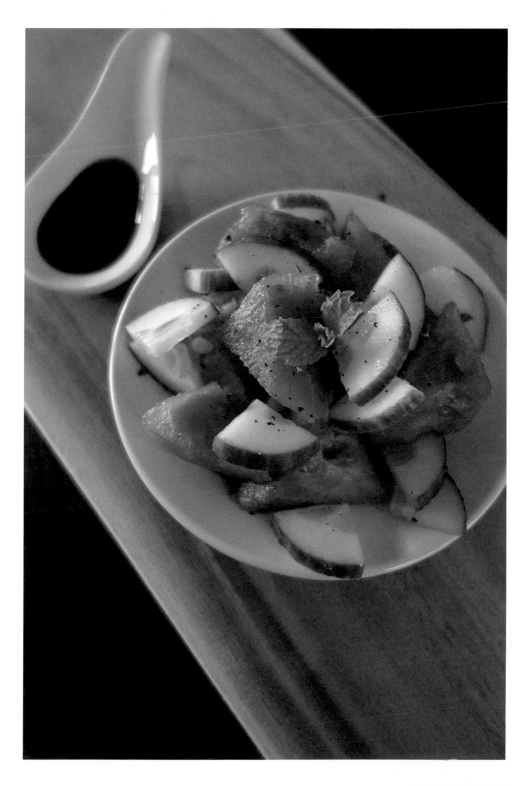

THE **YOUNG SKIN** DIET

DINNERS

ELASTICITY-BOOST ASIAN FUSION SALAD

DRESSING

½ cup extra virgin olive oil

⅙ cup apple cider vinegar

⅛ cup honey

1½ tbsp. fresh basil, chopped

1 garlic clove, crushed

⅛ tsp. salt

⅛ tsp. rosemary

Dash of red pepper flakes

CHICKEN

1 lb. dark meat chicken, cut into cubes

2 tsp. rosemary

¾ tsp. ground black pepper

Dash each of salt and red pepper flakes

SALAD

20 oz. spring mix greens

1 cup shredded carrots

40 cherry tomatoes, halved

1 cup unsalted cashews, toasted

Several slices of thinly cut red onion

Preheat oven to 350 degrees. As oven heats, whisk salad dressing ingredients together in a large bowl and set aside.

Mix chicken seasoning and rub onto meat, coating evenly.

Heat non-stick skillet over medium-high heat. Add a just enough olive oil to lightly coat the bottom of the skillet. Swirl to coat evenly.

Sauté chicken in skillet until cooked through, about 10 to 12 minutes. Meanwhile, place cashews on a non-stick cookie sheet and bake in oven for 3 to 5 minutes, until just starting to lightly brown.

Toss spring mix with desired amount of dressing, about 2 tbsp. per serving. Top with chicken, carrots, tomatoes, cashews, and red onion. Serve immediately.

Store leftover dressing in a tightly sealed glass jar and refrigerate. Shake before serving.

TIP For leftovers, store dressing, chicken and salad separately. Toss salad and chicken with dressing just before serving.

SCIENCE & NUTRITION

Olive Oil: Consumption of olive oil in the diet has been linked to reductions in the rate and severity of facial skin photoaging and to increased skin elasticity, with both effects leading to more youthful appearance.

- *Latreille, J., et al. "Dietary monounsaturated fatty acids intake and risk of skin photoaging," PLoS ONE. 2012 Sep.; 7(9): e44490.*

Apple Cider Vinegar: Vinegars, including apple cider vinegar, are associated with a host of nutritional benefits, including antioxidant and antimicrobial effects, which help reduce signs of aging.

- *Budak, N., et al. "Functional properties of vinegar," Journal of Food Science. 2014; 79(5): R757-R764.*

Spring Mix Greens + Carrot + Tomato: The phenolic and carotenoid antioxidants contained in vegetables including dark leafy greens, carrots and tomatoes exhibit synergistic effects that supercharge the radical-scavenging and anti-aging efforts of these foods when consumed in combination.

- *Milde, J., et al. "Synergistic effects of phenolics and carotenoids on human low-density lipoprotein oxidation," Molecular Nutrition and Food Research. 2007 Aug.; 51(8): 956-961.*

690 calories; 41g fat; 7g sat. fat; 76mg cholesterol; 200mg sodium; 1,680mg potassium; 45g carbohydrates; 7g fiber; 26g sugar; 39g protein. 5 servings.

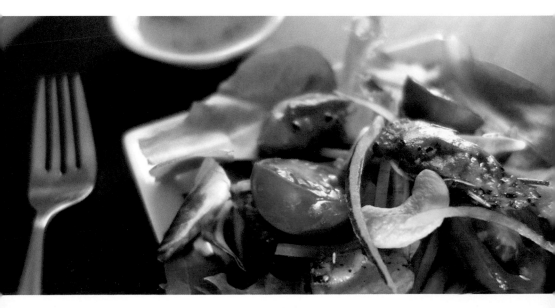

ERASE-THE-PHOTODAMAGE PRETTY POWERFUL PASTA

½ head of broccoli, chopped into bite-size florets

2 tbsp. extra virgin olive oil

2 garlic cloves, crushed

2 medium-sized, very ripe heirloom tomatoes, cored and chopped

3 anchovy fillets stored in extra virgin olive oil, chopped

8 oz. dry gluten-free quinoa fusilli pasta, prepared according to package instructions

Ground black pepper

Heat a small pot filled with ½ inch water over high heat. When water begins to boil, add broccoli, cover and cook for 2 minutes. Remove from heat, drain and set aside.

Heat olive oil in a non-stick skillet over medium to medium-high heat for 1 minute. Add garlic and stir until garlic is mixed into oil, being careful not to overcook.

Add broccoli, tomatoes and anchovies to skillet and sauté over medium-high heat for about 5 minutes, or until tomatoes have almost dissolved, broccoli has softened a bit and tomato-colored liquid has accumulated in the bottom of skillet.

Dish pasta into bowls and top with tomato, broccoli and anchovy mixture. Stir and season with freshly ground black pepper to taste.

SCIENCE & NUTRITION

Broccoli + Tomato + Olive Oil: Broccoli is rich in a flavonol called quercetin, which boasts powerful antioxidant and anti-inflammatory properties. The lycopene carotenoid in tomatoes can reduce the effects of UV photodamage on skin. Combined, the effects of broccoli and tomato are intensified. Plus, when tomatoes are cooked in olive oil, their lycopene molecules restructure to become more easily transmitted to skin tissue.

- *Vasanthi, H.R., et al. "Potential health benefits of broccoli – a chemico-biological overview," Mini-Reviews in Medicinal Chemistry. 2009 Jun.; 9(6): 749-759.*

- *Rizwan, M., et al. "Tomato paste rich in lycopene protects against cutaneous photodamage in humans in vivo: a randomized controlled trial" British Journal of Dermatology. 2011 Jan; 164(1): 154-162.*

- *Canene-Adams, K., et al. "Combinations of tomato and broccoli enhance antitumor activity in dunning r3327-h prostate adenocarcinomas," Cancer Research. 2007 Jan.; 67(2): 836-843.*

- *"Turning up the heat on tomatoes boosts absorption of lycopene," The Ohio State University Research News, Aug. 20, 2008: researchnews.osu.edu/archive/lycoproc.htm.*

Anchovies: The abundant Omega-3 fatty acids and very low mercury levels in anchovies make them an excellent source for nutrition that supports smooth and healthy skin.

- *Meschino, J.P. "Essential fatty acid supplementation improves skin texture and overall health," Dynamic Chiropractic. 2003 Sep.*

Quinoa: Phytoecdysteroids present in quinoa are powerful forces in preventing and delaying skin damage related to collagen loss and oxidative stress and thereby prolong skin's youthfulness.

• Nsimba, R.Y., et al. "Ecdysteroids act as inhibitors of calf skin collagenase and oxidative stress," Journal of Biochemical and Molecular Toxicology. 2008 Jul./Aug.; 22(4): 240-250.

390 calories; 12g fat; 2g sat. fat; 4mg cholesterol; 200mg sodium; 260mg potassium; 63g carbohydrates; 3g fiber; 3g sugar; 8g protein. 3 servings.

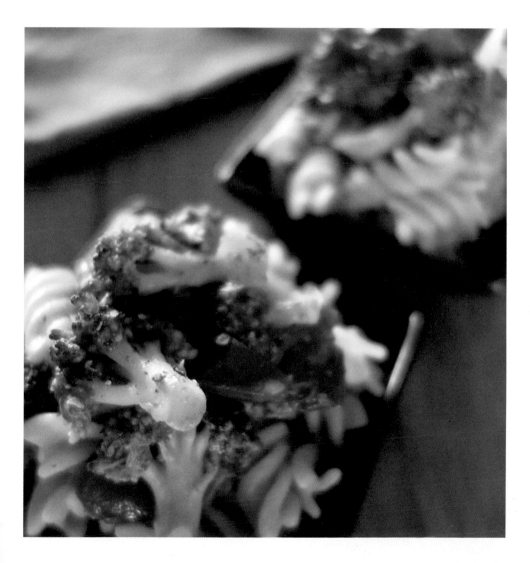

ANTI-WRINKLE SPICED SALMON & ASPARAGUS

SALMON

1 tsp. kosher salt or coarse sea salt

1 tsp. ground black pepper

½ tsp. cumin

½ tsp. coriander

½ tsp. allspice

1 lb. wild-caught salmon fillet (King salmon, particularly those from Alaska's Yukon River, contain the highest levels of Omega-3 fats and highest concentrations of DHA; Sockeye salmon also are a good choice for overall fat content), sliced into 4 oz. fillets and skinned

Extra virgin olive oil

1 lemon, quartered

ASPARAGUS

1 lb. asparagus spears, hard base snapped off

1 tbsp. extra virgin olive oil

¼ tsp. kosher salt or coarse sea salt

¼ tsp. coarse ground black pepper

Begin with salmon spices, mixing salt, pepper, cumin, coriander, and allspice in a small bowl. Sprinkle salmon to taste with spice mix.

Place salmon in a deep, non-stick skillet just large enough to fit fillets and pour olive into skillet until salmon is just covered. Sprinkle a little additional spice mix into skillet. Heat over low heat until oil reaches 130 degrees. Poach salmon at that temperature for 15 to 20 minutes or until salmon is tender and breaks apart with slight pressure.

While salmon cooks, fill a large, non-stick skillet with water and add a ¼ tsp. salt. Bring water to a simmer over medium heat. Add asparagus and cook for 2 to 3 minutes or until asparagus is bright green and tender.

Use tongs to remove asparagus from water. Dry with paper towel. Toss with olive oil, salt and pepper. Set aside.

When salmon is ready, remove salmon from oil. Blot with paper towel.

Drizzle fresh-squeezed lemon juice atop fillets and serve with asparagus on the side.

TIP For best results when poaching, look for salmon fillets that are relatively uniform in thickness.

SCIENCE & NUTRITION

Salmon: The animal-based Omega-3 fatty acids from fish are especially plentiful in salmon and impart potent anti-inflammatory effects that help improve skin condition and resistance to skin-related degradation from disease and aging. Long-chain Omega-3 fatty acids in salmon promote healthy skin that withstands environmental factors that result in aged appearance.

- *Boelsma, E., et al. "Nutritional skin care: health effects of micronutrients and fatty acids," The American Journal of Clinical Nutrition. 2001 May; 73(5): 853-864.*

Asparagus: A good source of vitamin K, asparagus has been shown to protect against skin wrinkling and to promote youthful appearance of skin.

- *Purba, M., et al. "Skin wrinkling: can food make a difference?" Journal of the American College of Nutrition. 2001; 20(1): 71-80.*

Salmon: 230 calories; 13g fat; 3g sat. fat; 72mg cholesterol; 500mg sodium; 530mg potassium; 1g carbohydrates; 0g fiber; 0g sugar; 28g protein. 4 servings.

Asparagus: 50 calories; 4g fat; 1g sat. fat; 0mg cholesterol; 110mg sodium; 230mg potassium; 5g carbohydrates; 2g fiber; 2g sugar; 2g protein. 4 servings.

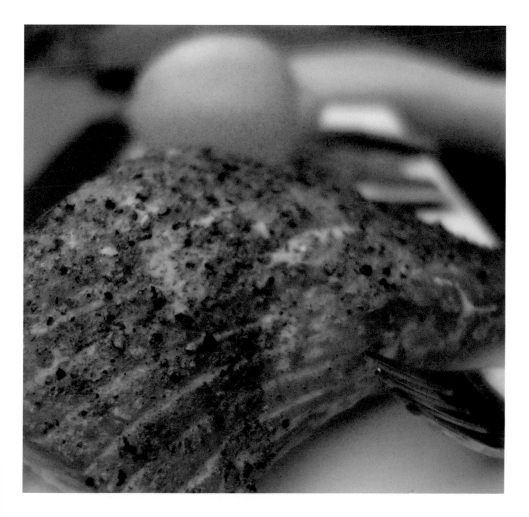

TONE 'N TEXTURE SHRIMP 'N VEGGIES

MARINADE

½ **cup extra virgin olive oil**

1 **tbsp. lemon juice**

3 **garlic cloves, minced**

1½ **tsp. salt**

1½ **tsp. honey**

¼ **tsp. ground black pepper**

VEGETABLE SKEWERS

2 **large, firm tomatoes, quartered**

2 **medium red onions, quartered**

2 **green peppers, cut into 1½-inch chunks**

10 **bamboo skewers, soaked in water 30 minutes**

1 **to 2 cups dry rice, prepared according to package instructions**

PROTEIN

1 **lb. wild caught shrimp, peeled and deveined (thawed if frozen)**

1 **lemon, quartered**

At least 4 hours prior to meal time, vigorously mix marinade ingredients in a small bowl. Place vegetables in a large, glass baking dish. Pour half of marinade over vegetables and toss to coat. Place shrimp in separate glass dish. Pour remaining marinade over shrimp. Cover both vegetables and shrimp with foil and refrigerate 4 to 8 hours.

Preheat broiler to high. Skewer vegetables.

Place vegetable skewers on broiler pan. Cook about 20 minutes or until onions and peppers are slightly browned and tomatoes almost fall off skewers. Rotate halfway through cooking time.

While vegetables cook, prepare rice according to package instructions. Then, place shrimp and marinade in a wide, shallow skillet. Turn heat to low, cover and poach until shrimp are pink and opaque, about 10 minutes. Shrimp are cooked when they form a "c" shape.

Remove shrimp from poaching liquid using a slotted spoon.

Serve shrimp and vegetables atop rice with lemon wedges for extra seasoning.

TIP For extra flavor, sprinkle shrimp with equal parts smoked paprika, garlic powder, chili powder, salt and pepper.

SCIENCE & NUTRITION

Shrimp: Containing astaxanthin and selenium, shrimp offer powerful skin-enhancing nutrients that improve skin tone and texture and enhance resistance to skin photoaging associated with UV exposure.

- *Pallela, R. "Antioxidants from marine organisms and skin care," Systems Biology of Free Radicals and Antioxidants. 2014 May; 166: 3771-3783.*

Red Onion: Onions, and especially red onions, exhibit strong antioxidant, anti-inflammatory and antibacterial effects, which collectively improve skin quality.

- *Wilson, E., et al. "Antioxidant, anti-inflammatory, and antimicrobial properties of garlic and onions," Nutrition & Food Science. 2007; 37(3): 178-183.*

300 calories; 5g fat; 1g sat. fat; 147mg cholesterol; 250mg sodium; 390mg potassium; 42g carbohydrates; 2g fiber; 6g sugar; 20g protein. 6 servings.

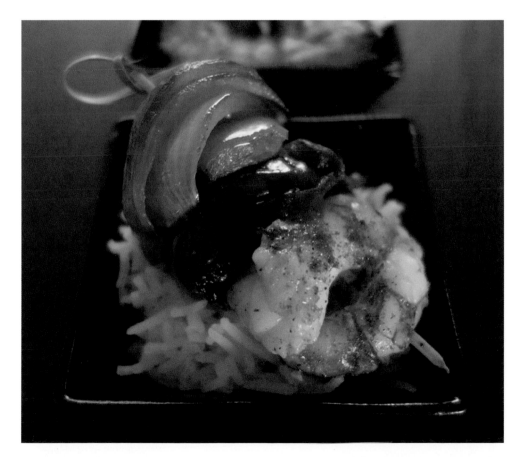

THE AGELESS MS. FIT BURGER

15 oz. canned black beans, drained, rinsed and mashed

2 medium beets, cooked, peeled and mashed

½ red bell pepper, chopped

¼ red onion chopped + ¼ red onion, thinly sliced

2 to 3 garlic cloves, minced

1 egg, lightly beaten

1 tsp. ground black pepper

1 tsp. smoked paprika

¼ tsp. salt

¼ to ½ cup cooked long grain white rice

1 to 2 tbsp. gluten-free oat flour

1 tbsp. unrefined coconut oil

Lettuce leaves

Combine mashed beans and beets in a large bowl. Set aside.

Place red pepper, chopped onion and garlic in a food processor and finely chop. Pour mixture into mashed beans and beets. Combine.

In a separate bowl, whisk together egg, black pepper, paprika and salt. Stir into bean mixture. Add rice and sliced onion and combine. Stir in oat flour, adding just enough to help mixture stick together.

Heat a large non-stick skillet over medium heat. Melt coconut oil in skillet and swirl to coat. Drop 6 patties onto skillet and use spatula to flatten.

Cook burgers until heated through, about 5 minutes per side. While burgers cook, sauté red onion in skillet alongside burgers.

Top burgers with sautéed onion. Serve wrapped in lettuce leaves.

SCIENCE & NUTRITION

Beet: The antioxidants in beets have been demonstrated to efficiently scavenge peroxyl and hydroxyl radicals, which can damage nucleic acids, amino acids and lipids in the body and skin and can lead to autoimmune diseases, all of which can contribute to an aged appearance.

- *Cao, G., et al. "Antioxidant capacity of tea and common vegetables," Journal of Agricultural and Food Chemistry. 1996 Nov.; 44(11): 3426-3431.*

Black Bean + Beet + Bell Pepper + Onion + Garlic: The antioxidant capacities of foods have been shown to exhibit greatest additive and synergistic effects when combined with foods from different food categories (e.g., as in this recipe, legumes with a root vegetable and three other vegetables).

- *Wang, S., et al. "Synergistic, additive, and antagonistic effects of food mixtures on total antioxidant capacities," Journal of Agricultural and Food Chemistry. 2011 Jan.; 59(3): 960-968.*

190 calories; 3g fat; 2g sat. fat; 36mg cholesterol; 200mg sodium; 150mg potassium; 31g carbohydrates; 5g fiber; 4g sugar; 8g protein. 6 servings.

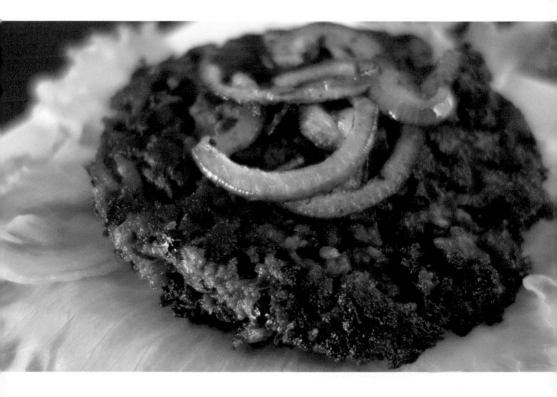

OMEGA-3 GARLIC BARRAMUNDI WITH MUSHROOMS & WILD RICE

1 cup dry wild rice, prepared according to package instructions

½ cup water

½ cup dry white wine or lemon juice

1 lb. barramundi, skinned and cut into 4 equal-sized fillets

2 tbsp. extra virgin olive oil for fish + 1 tbsp. for mushrooms

2 garlic cloves, minced or crushed

¼ tsp. sea salt

¼ tsp. ground black pepper

½ tsp. thyme

1 tsp. rosemary

8 oz. organic mushrooms, sliced

1 lemon, quartered

Pour water and wine (or lemon juice) into a large, non-stick skillet and place over medium heat for 5 minutes.

Slide barramundi fillets into poaching liquid, tops facing up. Top with 2 tbsp. olive oil and sprinkle with garlic, salt, pepper, thyme and rosemary.

Bring to a boil, reduce heat to medium, and poach until barramundi is firm and easily flakes with pressure, about 10 to 15 minutes.

While barramundi cooks, heat a large, non-stick skillet over medium heat. Add 1 tbsp. olive oil and swirl to coat. Sauté mushrooms in skillet until softened, about 5 to 10 minutes. Season to taste with salt and pepper.

Serve poached barramundi atop wild rice. Squeeze lemon juice over fillets and top with mushrooms.

TIP If fillets are thick in center, flip and poach for an additional 3 minutes or until centers are cooked through.

SCIENCE & NUTRITION

Barramundi + Olive Oil + Thyme + Rosemary: Also known as Asian Sea Bass, barramundi is usually available from aquaculture projects. Farmed barramundi exhibits excellent fatty acid characteristics, including high levels of Omega-3 fatty acids and a positive ratio of Omega-3 to Omega-6 fats, which benefits skin health. Herbs, including thyme and rosemary, stabilize fats and protect them from oxidation during cooking. Herbs accordingly enable the full health benefits of fish and extra virgin olive oil to be realized.

- Nichols, P., et al. "Readily available sources of long-chain omega-3 oils: is farmed Australian seafood a better source of the good oil than wild-caught seafood?" Nutrients. 2014; 6(3): 1063-1079.

- Uribarri, J., et al. "Advanced glycation end products in foods and a practical guide to their reduction in the the diet," Journal of the American Dietetic Association. 2010 Jun.; 110(6): 911-916.

Lemon + Rosemary: Citrus flavonoids from lemon and polyphenols and di-terpenes from rosemary have been shown to produce synergistic effects in protecting skin from photoaging, improving resistance to damage by as much as 56%. The field of protection encompasses keratinocyte cells, the primary cell type in skin's outer layer.

- *Perez-Sanchez, A., et al. "Protective effects of citrus and rosemary extracts on UV-in-duced damage in skin cell model and human volunteers," Journal of Photochemistry and Photobiology B: Biology. 2014 Jul.; 136: 12-18.*

400 calories; 16g fat; 2g sat. fat; 60mg cholesterol; 220mg sodium; 810mg potassium; 34g carbohydrates; 4g fiber; 1g sugar; 36g protein. 4 servings.

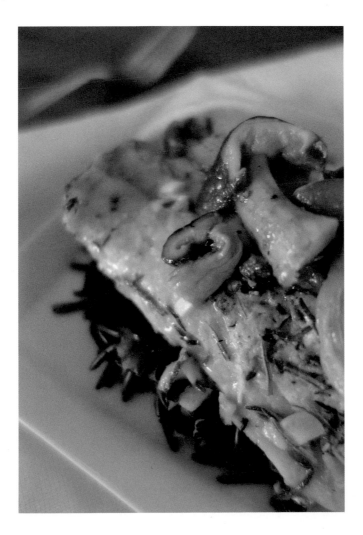

TIGHTEN-YOUR-SKIN SLOW COOKER YELLOW CURRY

2 lbs. skinless, boneless chicken breasts, cut into cubes

2 sweet potatoes, skin left on and cubed

1 red onion, chopped

1 garlic clove, minced

13.5 oz. coconut milk (full fat)

1 cup low sodium chicken broth

¼ cup curry powder

½ tsp. cinnamon

½ tsp. allspice

¼ tsp. salt

¼ tsp. ground black pepper

1 red bell pepper, chopped

½ cup green beans

1 tbsp. palm sugar

Coconut flakes (optional)

2 cups dry jasmine rice, prepared according to package instructions (optional)

Place chicken, potatoes, onion, garlic, coconut milk, chicken broth, curry powder, cinnamon, allspice, salt and black pepper in a slow cooker.

Cook on low for 4 hours. Add red bell pepper, green beans and palm sugar. Continue to cook on low for 45 minutes.

Serve plain or atop jasmine rice. Sprinkle with coconut flakes if desired.

SCIENCE & NUTRITION

Chicken + Garlic: Chicken is a good source of carnosine, which, like garlic, inhibits the formation of advanced glycation end products, precursors of skin aging. Carnosine and garlic are believed to work against advanced glycation end product formation through different mechanisms, suggesting that the concurrent consumption of both foods can result in superior results.

- *Danby, F.W. "Nutrition and aging skin: sugar and glycation," Clinics in Dermatology. 2010 Jul.-Aug.; 28(4): 409-411.*

Green Beans: Silicon is critical in skin health, as it is abundant in the collagen proteins found in the skin's intracellular matrix. Insufficient silicon levels are linked to reduced collagen levels and sagging, aged skin. While many plants contain silicon, not all is readily bioavailable to the body. Silicon found in green beans is both plentiful and bioavailable, ensuring the body absorbs and uses it in skin maintenance.

- *Sripanyakorn, S., et al. "The comparative absorption of silicon from different foods and food supplements," British Journal of Nutrition. 2009 Sep.; 102(6): 825-834.*

540 calories; 19g fat; 12g sat. fat; 96mg cholesterol; 210mg sodium; 590mg potassium; 49g carbohydrates; 2g fiber; 5g sugar; 39g protein. 8 servings.

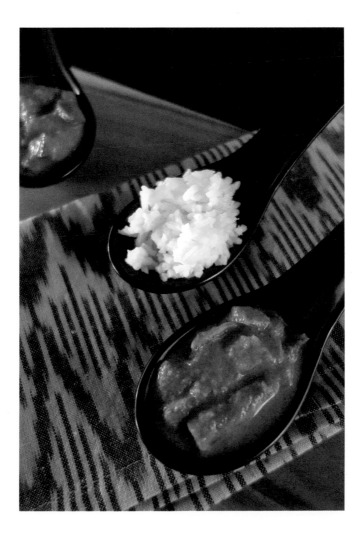

THE **YOUNG SKIN** DIET

DESSERTS

RESTORATIVE HOT HONEY FRUIT

2 tsp. fresh-squeezed lime juice	Mix lime and honey together in a small bowl and set aside.
2 tsp. honey	Divide fruit into two serving bowls. Drizzle with honey-lime mixture, add a pinch of cayenne pepper and serve.
15 to 20 blueberries	
7 to 10 blackberries	
4 to 5 strawberries, sliced	
1 orange	
Cayenne pepper	

SCIENCE & NUTRITION

Blueberries + Blackberries + Strawberries: Every type of berry (and fruit, generally) contains a rich diversity of phytochemicals, which provide antioxidant effects. When different types of berries are combined, their individual antioxidant activities are magnified, powerfully erasing precursors of skin aging and maintaining healthy skin cell function.

- *Seeram, N., et al. Antioxidant Measurement and Applications. ACS Symposium Series, Vol. 956, 2009: Chapter 21: "Impact of berry phytochemicals on human health: effects beyond antioxidation."*

Cayenne Pepper: Capsaicin is a strong anti-inflammatory agent that promotes healthy skin. It is also a natural analgesic that assists in rest and sleeping, so the body's own restorative capacities can be tapped during the sleep cycle.

- *Kim, C. "Capsaicin exhibits anti-inflammatory property by inhibiting IkB-a degradation in LPS-stimulated peritoneal macrophages," Cell Signal. 2003 Mar.; 15(3): 299-306.*

90 calories; 0g fat; 0g sat. fat; 0mg cholesterol; 0mg sodium; 230mg potassium; 22g carbohydrates; 4g fiber; 18g sugar; 1g protein. 2 servings.

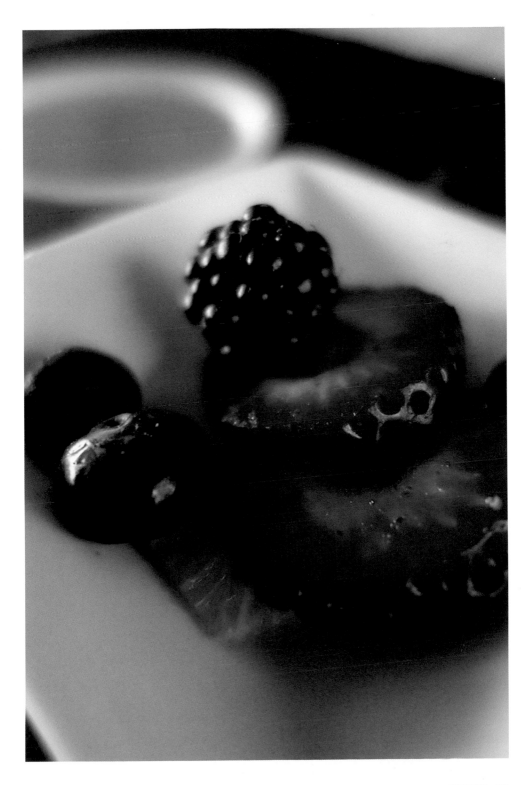

UV PROTECTION CITRUS SALAD

1 orange, peeled and segmented + ½ tsp. orange zest

1 grapefruit, peeled and segmented

1 kiwi, peeled and chopped

Mix fruit together in a bowl, sprinkle with orange zest and enjoy.

TIP Try using a blood orange or cara cara orange if in season.

SCIENCE & NUTRITION

Grapefruit + Orange: The carotenoids and flavonoids in citrus fruits have been shown to prevent UV damage in human skin. Synergies among the compounds of citrus fruits suggest consuming different citrus varieties simultaneously magnifies their protective effects.

- *Stahl, W., et al. "Carotenoids and flavonoids contribute to nutritional protection against skin damage from sunlight," Molecular Biology. 2007 Sep.; 37(1): 26-30.*
- *Grosso, G., et al. "Red orange: experimental models and epidemiological evidence of its benefits on human health," Oxidative Medicine and Cellular Longevity. 2013: 1-11.*
- *McClain, G., et al. "The role of polyphenols in skin health," Bioactive Dietary Factors and Plant Extracts in Dermatology Nutrition and Health. 2013: 169-175.*

Kiwi + Grapefruit + Orange: The zinc in kiwi is an essential mineral that promotes healthy skin, hair, nails and teeth. Citrate, a form of ascorbic acid found in citrus fruits, enhances the body's absorption of zinc, thus enabling full utilization of kiwi's mineral content. Grapefruit is one of the richest sources of citrate.

- *Chasapis, C, et al. "Zinc and human health: an update," Archives of Toxicology. 2012 Apr.; 86(4): 521-534.*
- *Lonnerdal, B. "Dietary factors influencing zinc absorption," The Journal of Nutrition. 2000 May; 130(5): 1378S-1383S.*
- *Haleblian, G.E., et al. "Assessment of citrate concentrates in citrus fruit-based juices and beverages: implications for management of hypocitraturic nephrolithiasis," Journal of Endourology. 2008 Jun.; 22(6): 1359-1366.*

100 calories; 0g fat; 0g sat. fat; 0mg cholesterol; 0mg sodium; 390mg potassium; 26g carbohydrates; 5g fiber; 17g sugar; 2g protein. 2 servings.

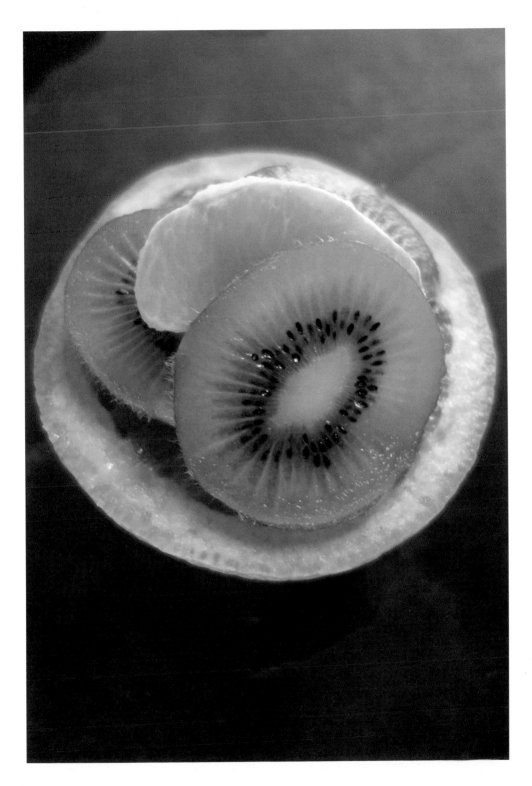

CELLULAR REPAIR FIGS WITH WALNUTS & HONEY

½ **tbsp. unrefined coconut oil**

10 fresh figs, halved lengthwise

½ **tsp. palm sugar**

¼ **cup walnut pieces, unsalted**

Honey

Preheat oven to 400 degrees and line a baking sheet with foil.

"Butter" cut side of figs with coconut oil and sprinkle with palm sugar.

Place figs buttered/sugared side down on baking sheet. Bake until figs are soft and browned on the bottom, about 10 to 15 minutes.

When figs have 3 to 5 minutes left, place walnuts on baking sheet and continue baking. Walnuts should bake until they turn slightly golden brown on the outside.

Place figs and walnuts in serving bowls and drizzle with honey. Serve.

SCIENCE & NUTRITION

Figs: As part of the traditional Mediterranean diet, figs are powerful contributors of antioxidants, including polyphenols and anthocyanins.

- *Solomon, A. "Antioxidant activities and anthocyanin content of fresh fruits of common fig (ficus carica l.)," Journal of Agricultural and Food Chemistry. 2006; 54(20): 7717-7723.*

Walnuts: Walnuts contribute healthy fats as well as antioxidants. The melatonin found in walnuts increases the antioxidant capacity of the blood, thus enhancing cellular health in the body, including skin.

- *Reiter, R., et al. "Melatonin in walnuts: influence on levels of melatonin and total antioxidant capacity of blood," Nutrition. 2005 Sep.; 21(9): 920-924.–*

200 calories; 11g fat; 3g sat. fat; 0mg cholesterol; 0mg sodium; 350mg potassium; 29g carbohydrates; 4g fiber; 22g sugar; 2g protein. 4 servings.

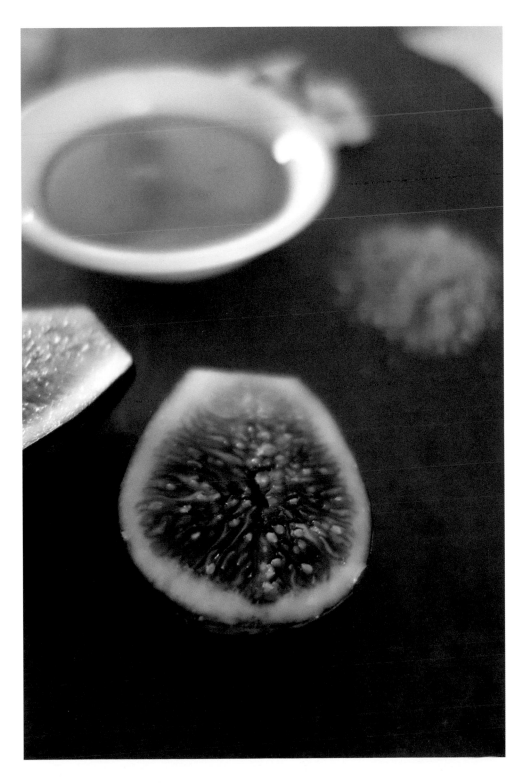

SUPER ANTIOXIDANT ALLSPICE MANGO

½ **ripe mango, peeled and pit removed**

Quatre épices spice mix (¼ tsp. allspice, ¼ tsp. nutmeg, ¼ tsp. cinnamon, and dash of cloves)

Arrange mango slices in bowl and sprinkle with quatre épices mix. Serve.

SCIENCE & NUTRITION

Mango: Mangiferin, which is found only in mango and a couple of other exotic plants, is among the most potent of antioxidants and has been referred to as a "super antioxidant." Mangiferin is abundant in mangoes and fights oxidation, cancer, inflammation, infection, allergy and pain, providing the body with system-wide benefits that health support healthy, youthful skin.

- *Masibo, M., et al. "Major mango polyphenols and their potential significance to human health," Comprehensive Reviews in Food Science and Food Safety. 2008 Oct.; 7(4): 309-319.*

Allspice: The antioxidant activity of allspice has been shown to enhance overall metabolic function that supports processes including collagen production in the skin.

- *Kochhar, K.P. "Dietary spices in health and diseases: I," Indian Journal of Physiology and Pharmacology. 2008 Apr.-Jun.; 52(2): 106-122.*

100 calories; 1g fat; 0g sat. fat; 0mg cholesterol; 0mg sodium; 280mg potassium; 25g carbohydrates; 3g fiber; 23g sugar; 2g protein. 1 serving.

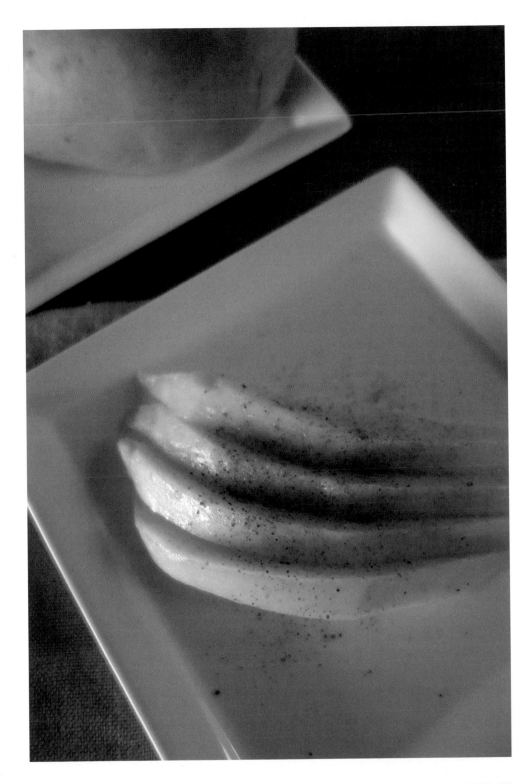

REVERSE-THE-CLOCK PISTACHIO & HONEY

¼ cup pistachios, roughly chopped

Honey

Cinnamon

Clove

Nutmeg

Place pistachios in a small bowl and drizzle with honey. Sprinkle with cinnamon, clove and nutmeg. Serve.

TIP For extra texture and flavor, serve over warm, sliced apples.

SCIENCE & NUTRITION

Clove + Nutmeg: Clove contains one of the highest concentrations of antioxidants, conferring protection against an array of environmental and chronological factors associated with skin aging. Nutmeg also provides plentiful natural antioxidants with excellent radical scavenging capabilities that protect health and support healthy skin. (Note that clove and nutmeg, if consumed at very high levels, may have deleterious health consequences. The spice should accordingly be used in moderation.)

- Shan, B., et al. "Antioxidant capacity of 26 spice extracts and characterization of their phenolic constituents," Journal of Agricultural and Food Chemistry. 2005 Sep.; 53(20): 7749-7759.

- Su, L., et al. "Total phenolic contents, chelating capacities, and radical-scavenging properties of black peppercorn, nutmeg, rosehip, cinnamon and oregano leaf," Food Chemistry. 2007; 100(3): 990-997.

210 calories; 14g fat; 2g sat. fat; 0mg cholesterol; 0mg sodium; 320mg potassium; 20g carbohydrates; 3g fiber; 13g sugar; 6g protein. 1 serving.

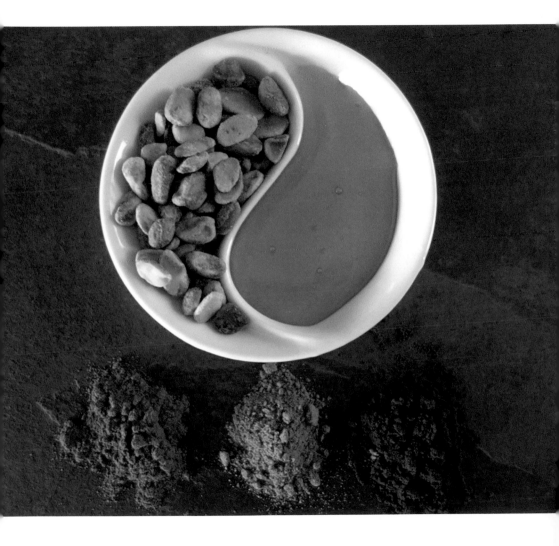

AGE-DEFYING TROPICAL FRUIT DESSERT

¼ **cup cantaloupe, cubed**

¼ **cup honeydew, cubed**

1 tbsp. pumpkin seeds, finely chopped

Combine cantaloupe and honeydew cubes in bowl.

Sprinkle with chopped pumpkin seeds. Serve.

SCIENCE & NUTRITION

Cantaloupe: Beta-carotene, the plant-derived form of vitamin A most readily used by the human body, is abundant in cantaloupes. Intake of beta-carotene has been shown to improve facial wrinkles, skin elasticity, enhance collagen production and reduce skin pigmentation 'staining' from UV damage.

- *Cho, S., et al. "The role of functional foods in cutaneous anti-aging," Journal of Lifestyle Medicine. 2014 Mar.; 4(1): 8-16.*
- *Cho, S., et al. "Differential effects of low-dose and high-dose beta-carotene supplementation on the signs of photo-aging and type I procollagen gene expression in human skin in vivo," Dermatology. 2010; 221: 160-171.*

Cantaloupe + Honeydew + Pumpkin Seeds: The beta-carotene (from cantaloupe), the vitamin C (from honeydew), and the vitamin E (from pumpkin seeds) interact synergistically to scavenge radicals from the body and provide strong antioxidant and anti-aging benefits in the skin.

- *Niki, E., et al. "Ineraction among vitamin C, vitamin E, and beta-carotene." American Journal of Clinical Nutrition. 1995 Dec.; 62(6 Supp.): 1322S-1326S.*

Pumpkin Seeds: The tocopherols (including the vitamin E tocopherol) in pumpkin seeds exhibit broad diversity that implies significant antioxidant benefits for human health, including human skin, as a result of postulated additive and synergistic activity among the tocopherols. The diversity of tocopherol antioxidants in pumpkin seeds is uniquely broad.

- *Stevenson, D., et al. "Oil and tocopherol content and composition of pumpkin seed oil in 12 cultivars," Journal of Agricultural and Food Chemistry. 2007; 55(10): 4005-4013.*

150 calories; 1g fat; 0g sat. fat; 0mg cholesterol; 70mg sodium; 980mg potassium; 36g carbohydrates; 4g fiber; 31g sugar; 3g protein. 1 serving.

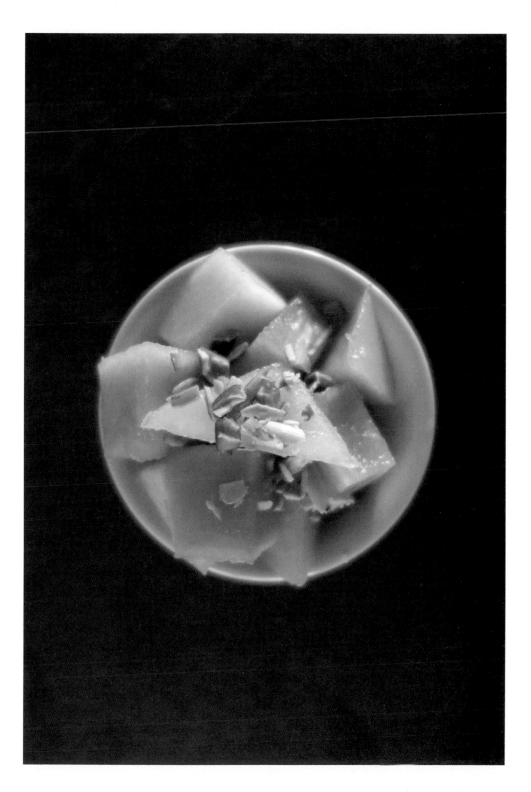

SWEET DREAMS SMOOTHIE

1 banana | Place ingredients in blender. Blend until smooth.
½ cup frozen cherries | Enjoy and sleep tight!
¼ cup coconut milk |

SCIENCE & NUTRITION

Cherry + Banana: Melatonin, an antioxidant abundant in cherries, plays an important role in human sleep regulation. Consumption of melatonin-rich cherries increases blood melatonin levels and promotes improved sleep, which allows the body's natural skin healing mechanisms time and resources to perform optimally. Bananas contain tryptophan and serotonin (serotonin also is present in cherries), which promote sleep and feelings of well-being, respectively. Combined with the melatonin, tryptophan and serotonin work to ensure deep, restful and restorative sleep.

- *Howatson, G., et al. "Effects of tart cherry juice (prunus cerasus) on melatonin levels and enhanced sleep quality," European Journal of Nutrition. 2012 Dec.; 51(8): 909-916.*

- *Gonzalez-Gomez, D., et al. "Detection and quantification of melatonin and serotonin in eight sweet cherry cultivars (prunus avium l.)," European Food Research and Technology. 2009 Jun.; 229(2): 223-229.*

- *Ohla, S., et al. "Chip electrophoresis of active banana ingredients with label-free detection utilizing deep UV native fluorescence and mass spectrometry," Analytical and Bioanalytical Chemistry. 2011 Feb.; 339(5): 1853-1857.*

240 calories; 12g fat; 11g sat. fat; 0mg cholesterol; 20mg sodium; 630mg potassium; 35g carbohydrates; 4g fiber; 19g sugar; 3g protein. 1 serving

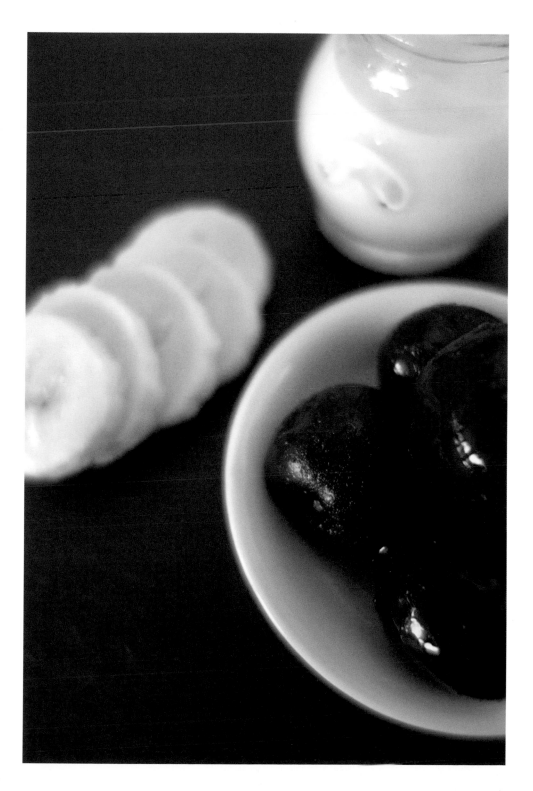

THE **YOUNG SKIN** DIET

SKIN TREATMENTS

SKIN-BRIGHTENING COCONUT OIL EXFOLIANT

1 tsp. unrefined coconut oil

1 tsp. fresh-squeezed lemon juice

1 tsp. granulated cane sugar

If coconut oil is solid, heat in microwave until just liquefied but not hot. Squeeze lemon into small bowl and mix juice with oil. Add sugar and stir.

Remove dirt and makeup from face. Coat hands, face and neck with mixture, rubbing lightly to exfoliate. Exfoliate for 2 to 3 minutes and then let mask rest for 7 to 10 minutes. Wash with regular face wash and warm water. Apply normal moisturizer and sunscreen.

TIP Lemon may increase skin's sensitivity to sun. For best results, apply mask before bedtime. Wear sunscreen and a hat during the day to prevent unnecessary sun exposure.

SCIENCE

Coconut Oil: Topical application of coconut oil has been linked with increased hydration and elasticity of skin, with usage resulting in hydration and elasticity levels more than 140% those of untreated skin immediately following application. Hydration and elasticity improvement grows to 175% after 3 weeks of regular usage. Compared with lotions not including coconut oil's fats and phytochemicals, coconut oil treatments result in more than 3 times the skin elasticity improvements. Unrefined virgin coconut oil also contains phenolic compounds that act as antioxidants.

- *Kapoor, S. and S. Saraf. "Assessment of viscoelasticity and hydration effect of herbal moisturizers using bioengineering techniques," Pharmacognosy Magazine. 2010 Oct.-Dec.; 6(24): 298-304.*

- *Noor, N.M, et al. "The effect of virgin coconut oil loaded solid lipid particles (VCO-SLPs) on skin hydration and skin elasticity," Journal Teknologi. 2013 May; 62(1): 39-43.*

- *Marina, A.M., et al. "Antioxidant capacity and phenolic acids of virgin coconut oil," International Journal of Food Sciences and Nutrition. 2009; 60(Supp. 2): 114-123.*

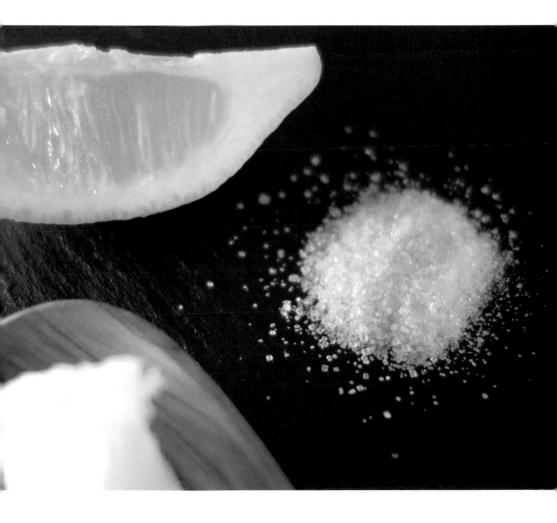

CALM SKIN TURMERIC MASK

2 tsp. honey	Mix ingredients in a small bowl to create a paste.
1 tsp. turmeric	Remove dirt and makeup from face. Coat hands, face and neck with mixture. Let mask rest for 7 to 10 minutes. Wash skin with warm water and regular face wash. Apply normal moisturizer and sunscreen.
	TIP Turmeric may temporarily turn skin slightly yellow. Washing with regular face wash should remove residual color. Unrefined coconut oil or olive oil may also be used to remove any remaining color.

SCIENCE

Turmeric: Compounds in turmeric, including curcumin, exhibit strong anti-inflammatory effects that calm the skin and enhance youthful appearance.

- *Epstein, J., et al. "Curcumin as therapeutic agent: the evidence from in vitro, animal and human studies," British Journal of Nutrition. 2010 Jun.; 103(11): 1545-1557.*

- *Lantz, R., et al. "The effect of turmeric extracts on inflammatory mediator production," Phytomedicine. 2005 Jun.; 12(6-7): 445-452.*

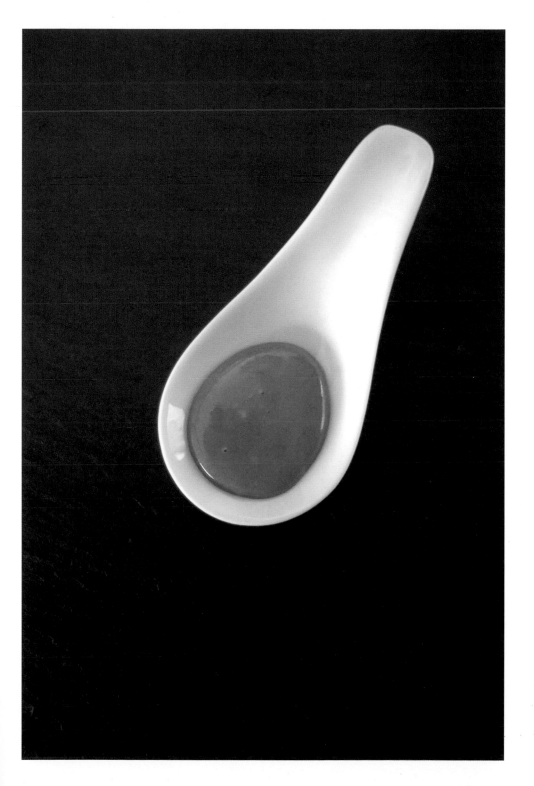

ELIMINATE-FREE-RADICALS OLIVE OIL & GINGER BATH

2 tsp. extra virgin olive oil

1 tsp. finely ground or smashed fresh ginger root

Mix ingredients in a small bowl.

Remove dirt and makeup from face. Coat hands, face and neck with bath. Let rest for 7 to 10 minutes. Rinse skin with warm water. Once most of oil has been removed, wash with regular face wash and warm water. Apply normal moisturizer and sunscreen.

SCIENCE

Olive oil: Application of olive oil to the skin can help reduce UV-induced damage due to the ability of olive oil phenols caffeic acid and ferulic acid to permeate the skin and scavenge free radicals.

- *Saija, A., et al. "In vitro and in vivo evaluation of caffeic and ferulic acids as topical photoprotective agents," International Journal of Pharmaceutics. 2000 Apr.; 199(1): 39-47.*

- *Ghanbari, R., et al. "Valuable nutrients and functional bioactives in different parts of olive (olea europea l.) – a review," International Journal of Molecular Sciences. 2012; 13(3): 3291-3340.*

Ginger: Topical application of ginger can reduce skin inflammation, thus calming skin's appearance and enhancing youthfulness.

- *Sosa, M., et al. "Evaluation of the topical anti-inflammatory activity of ginger dry extracts from solutions and plasters," Planta Medica. 2007; 73(15): 1525-1530.*

- *Shukla, Y., et al. "Cancer preventive properties of ginger: a brief review," Food and Chemical Toxicology. 2007 May; 45(5): 683-690.*

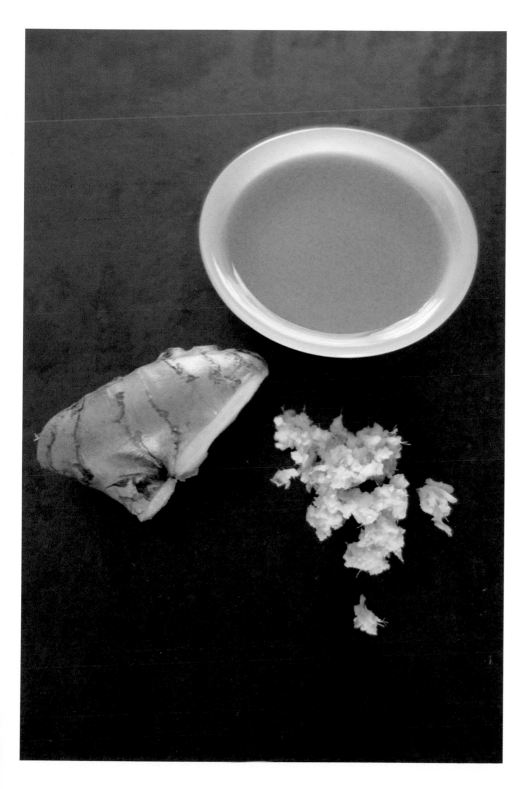

LEMON WATER & CANE SUGAR SKIN TONING MASK

1 tsp. fresh-squeezed lemon juice

1 tsp. granulated cane sugar

Mix ingredients in a small bowl.

Remove dirt and makeup from face. Coat hands, face and neck with mixture, rubbing very lightly in a circular motion. (Do not rub too hard, or sugar granules can injure skin.) Let mask rest for 7 to 10 minutes. Rinse skin with lukewarm water, wash face with regular face wash, and apply normal moisturizer and sunscreen.

TIP Lemon may increase skin's sensitivity to sun. For best results, apply mask before bedtime. Wear sunscreen and a hat during the day to prevent unnecessary sun exposure.

SCIENCE

Lemon Juice + Cane Sugar: Lemon contains citric acid and cane sugar contains glycolic acid. Both citric acid and glycolic acid are alpha-hydroxy acid chemexfoliants that have been shown to reverse photoaging damage in human skin, including problems relating to pigmentation and collagen loss.

- *Yamamoto, Y., et al. "Effects of alpha-hydroxy acids on the human skin of Japanese subjects: the rationale for chemical peeling," Journal of Dermatology. 2006 Jan.; 33(1): 16-22.*

- *Ditre, C. "Glycolic acid peels," Dermatologic Therapy. 2000 Apr.; 13(2): 165-172.*

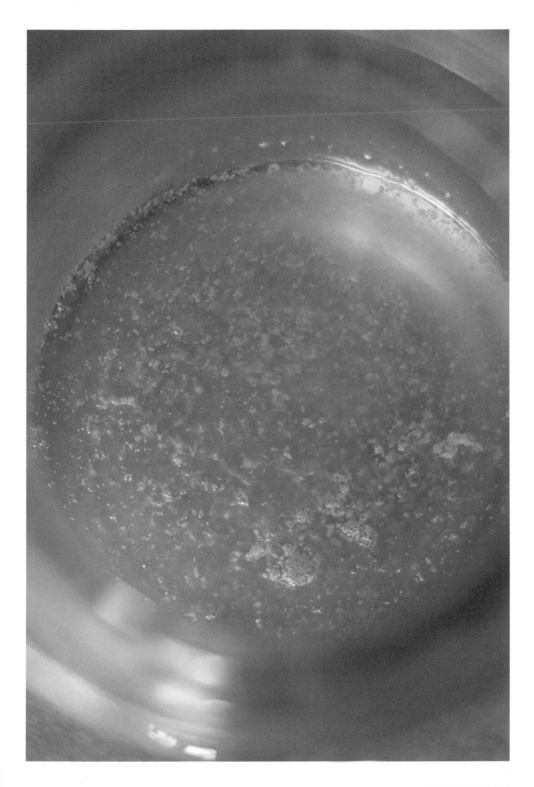

NO-MORE-INFLAMMATION HONEY & OLIVE OIL MASK

1 tsp. honey	Mix ingredients in a small bowl.
1 tsp. extra virgin olive oil	Remove dirt and makeup from face. Coat hands, face and neck with mixture. Let mask rest for 7 to 10 minutes. Wash with regular face wash and apply normal moisturizer and sunscreen.

SCIENCE

Honey + Olive Oil: When applied topically to skin, a mixture of honey and olive oil has been shown effective at reducing inflammation and the redness and dryness associated with atopic dermatitis/eczema and psoriasis, implying a role in reducing skin inflammation and improving tone in otherwise healthy individuals. Honey and olive oil-based moisturizer treatments also are associated with skin hydration and skin elasticity improvements of more than 60%.

- *Al-Waili, N.S. "Topical application of natural honey, beeswax and olive oil mixture for atopic dermatitis or psoriasis: partially controlled, single-blinded study," Complementary Therapies in Medicine. 2003 Dec.; 11(4): 226-234.*

- *Kapoor, S. and S. Saraf. "Assessment of viscoelasticity and hydration effect of herbal moisturizers using bioengineering techniques," Pharmacognosy Magazine. 2010 Oct.-Dec.; 6(24): 298-304.*

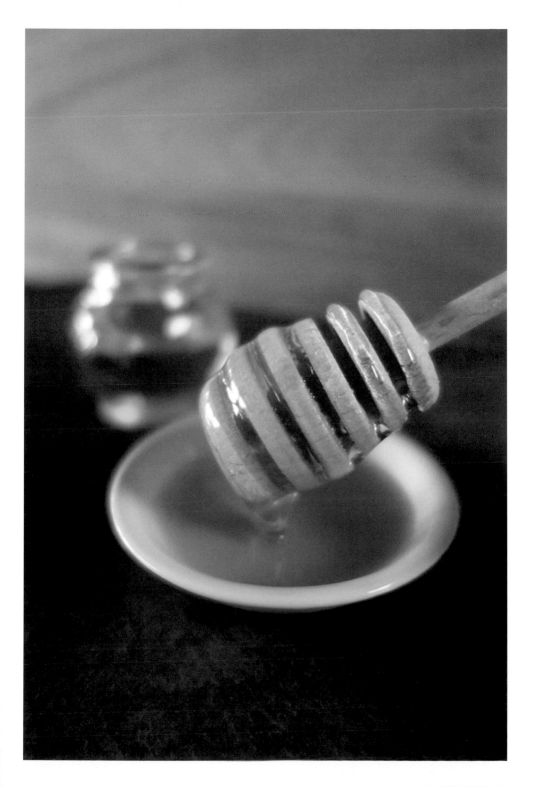

UV DAMAGE-REDUCING GREEN TEA MASK

1 sachet green tea	Make tea according to package instructions.
8 oz. water	Remove dirt and makeup from face. Use tea bag to apply green tea to face and neck, dabbing onto skin until skin is moist. Let mask rest for 7 to 10 minutes. Wash with regular face wash and apply normal moisturizer and sunscreen.

SCIENCE

Green Tea: Polyphenolic antioxidants in green tea provide skin photoprotection and enhance skin structure and function, protecting against wrinkle formation, melanin hyperpigmentation and cancer. Green tea applications to skin can resolve UV-related aging.

- *Heinrich, U., et al. "Green tea polyphenols provide photoprotection, increase microcirculation, and modulate skin properties of women," The Journal of Nutrition. 2011 Jun.; 141(6): 1202-1208.*

- *Roh, E., et al. "Molecular mechanisms of green tea polyphenols with protective effects against skin photoaging," Critical Reviews in Food Science and Nutrition. 2015.*

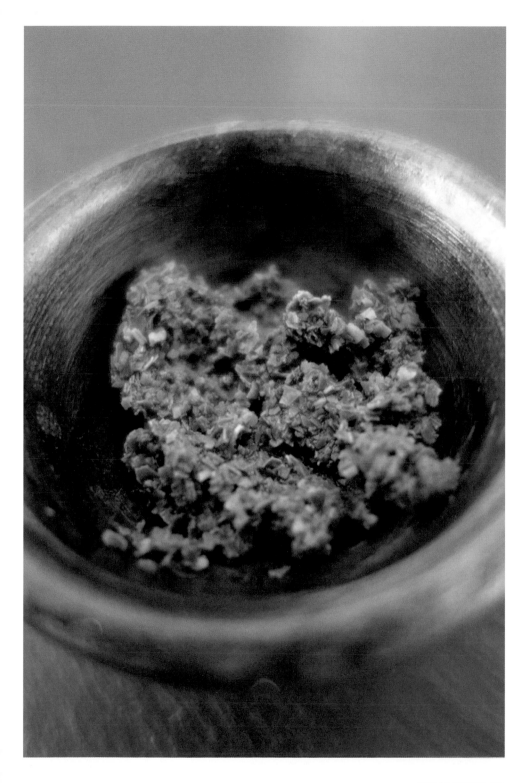

NO-MORE-IRRITATION CUCUMBER TREATMENT

1 medium towel, dampened with filtered water

Heat towel in microwave until warm, about 30 seconds to 1 minute.

½ cucumber, sliced into ¼-inch rounds

Remove dirt and makeup from face. Wrap warm towel over face, leaving openings at eyes and mouth. Lie down. Place cucumber rounds over eyes, at hairline and at corners of mouth. Place two cucumber rounds on the back of each hand. Leave treatment in place for 7 to 10 minutes.

Remove treatment and rinse face with warm water. Apply normal moisturizer and sunscreen.

SCIENCE

Warm Towel: A warm towel compress enhances skin elasticity and improves blood circulation through capillaries feeding the skin.

- *Jolly, H., et al. "Impact of warm compresses on local injection-site reactions with self-administered glatiramer acetate," Journal of Neuroscience Nursing. 2008 Aug.; 40(4): 232-240.*

Cucumber: Topical application of cucumber has been shown to reduce skin irritation, enhance wound healing, and improve new tissue growth by virtue of cucumber's antioxidant and flavonoid content.

- *Patil, M., et al. "Pharmacological evaluation of ameliorative effect of aqueous extract of cucumis sativus l. fruit formulation on wound healing in wistar rats," Chronicles of Young Scientists. 2011; 2(4): 207-213.*

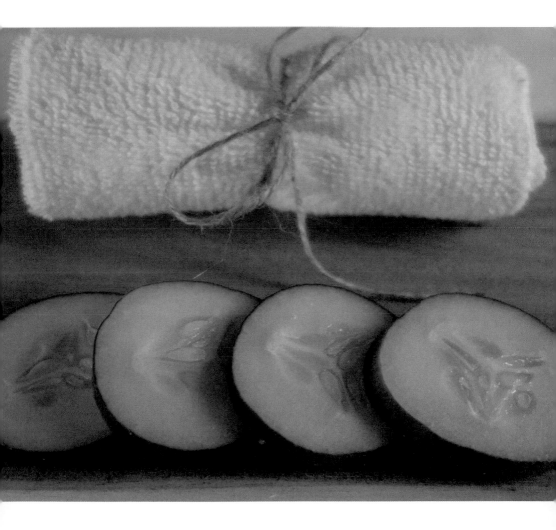

INGREDIENT INDEX

RESEARCH REFERENCES & FURTHER READING

Abugoch, J. "Quinoa (chenopodium quinoa willd.): composition, chemistry, nutritional, and functional properties," Advances in Food and Nutrition Research. 2009; 58: 1-31.

Akramiene, D., et al. "Effects of beta-glucans on the immune system," Medicina. 2007; 43(8): 597-606.

Al-Waili, N.S. "Topical application of natural honey, beeswax and olive oil mixture for atopic dermatitis or psoriasis: partially controlled, single-blinded study," Complementary Therapies in Medicine. 2003 Dec.; 11(4): 226-234.

Ananingsih, V., et al. "Green tea catechins during food processing and storage: a review on stability and detection," Food Research International. 2013 Mar.; 50(2): 469-479.

Ankri, S., et al. "Antimicrobial properties of allicin from garlic," Microbes and Infection. 1999 Feb.; 1(2): 125-129.

Applegate, E. "Introduction: nutritional and functional roles of eggs in the diet," Journal of the American College of Nutrition. 2000; 19(Supp. 5): 495S-498S.

Aruna G., et al. "Combined effect of ginger and honey against salmonellosis," Global Journal for Research Analysis. 2014 Aug.; 3(8): 1-3.

Aseervatham, G., et al. "Environmental factors and unhealthy lifestyle influence oxidative stress in humans—an overview," Environmental Science and Pollution Research. 2013 Jul.; 20(7): 4356-4369.

Balakrishnan, K.P., et al. "Botanicals as sunscreens: their role in the prevention of photoaging and skin cancer," International Journal of Research in Cosmetic Science. 2011; 1(1): 1-12.

Barcelo-Coblijn, G., et al. "Alpha-linolenic acid and its conversion to longer chain n-3 fatty acids: benefits for human health and a role in maintaining tissue n-3 fatty acid levels," Progress in Lipid Research. 2009 Nov.; 48(6): 355-374.

Barel, A., et al. "Effect of oral intake of choline-stabilized orthosilicic acid on skin, nails and hair of women with photodamaged skin," Archives of Dermatological Research. 2005 Oct.; 297(4): 147-153.

Bhaskaran, N., et al. "Chamomile: An anti-inflammatory agent inhibits inducible nitric oxide synthase expression by blocking RelA/p65 activity," International Journal of Molecular Medicine. 2010 Dec.; 26(6): 935-940.

Blanpain, C. and E. Fuchs. "Epidermal stem cells of the skin," Annual Review of Cell and Developmental Biology. 2006; 22: 339-373.

Blanpain, C., et al. "Self-renewal, multipotency, and the existence of two cell populations within an epithelial stem cell niche," Cell. 2004 Sept., 118: 625-648.

Boelsma, E., et al. "Nutritional skin care: health effects of micronutrients and fatty acids," The American Journal of Clinical Nutrition. 2001 May; 73(5): 853-864.

Boyer, J., et al. "Apple phytochemicals and their health benefits," Nutrition Journal. 2004; 3: 5-21.

Boyern N., et al. "Effect of vitamin C and its derivatives on collagen synthesis and cross-linking by normal human fibroblasts," International Journal of Cosmetic Science. 1998 Jun.; 20(3): 151-158.

Brufau, G., et al. "Nuts: source of energy and macronutrients," British Journal of Nutrition. 2006 Nov.; 96(Supp. 2): S22-S28.

Budak, N., et al. "Functional properties of vinegar," Journal of Food Science. 2014; 79(5): R757-R764.

Candela, C., et al. "Importance of balanced omega 6/omega 3 ratio for the maintenance of health," Nutrition Hospital. 2011; 26(2): 323-329.

Canene-Adams, K., et al. "Combinations of tomato and broccoli enhance antitumor activity in dunning r3327-h protstate adenocarcinomas," Cancer Research. 2007 Jan.; 67(2): 836-843.

Cao, G., et al. "Antioxidant capacity of tea and common vegetables," Journal of Agricultural and Food Chemistry. 1996 Nov.; 44(11): 3426-3431.

Caponio, F. et al., "Fatty acid composition and degradation level of the oils used in canned fish as a function of the different types of fish," Journal of Food Composition and Analysis. 2011 Dec.; 24(8): 1117-1122.

Chandrasekara, N., et al. "Effect of roasting on phenolic content and antioxidant activities of whole cashew nuts, kernels, and testa," Journal of Agricultural and Food Chemistry. 2011; 59(9): 5006-5014.

Chasapis, C, et al. "Zinc and human health: an update," Archives of Toxicology. 2012 Apr.; 86(4): 521-534.

Chawla, S., et al. "Overview of mint (mentha l.) as a promising health-promoting herb," International Journal of Pharmaceutical Research and Development. 2013 Aug.; 5(6): 73-80.

Chen, G. and J. Smith, "Determination of advanced glycation endproducts in cooked meat products," Food Chemistry. 2015 Feb.; 168(1): 190-195.

Chen, W., et al. "Functions of hyaluronan in wound repair," Wound Repair and Regeneration. 1999 Mar.-Apr.; 7(2): 79-89.

Cho, S., et al. "Differential effects of low-dose and high-dose beta-carotene supplementation on the signs of photo-aging and type I procollagen gene expression in human skin in vivo," Dermatology. 2010; 221: 160-171.

Cho, S., et al. "The role of functional foods in cutaneous anti-aging," Journal of Lifestyle Medicine. 2014 Mar.; 4(1): 8-16.

Chung, K., et al. "Tannins and human health: a review," Critical Reviews in Food Science and Nutrition. 1998 Aug.; 38(6): 421-464.

Collins, J., et al. "Watermelon consumption increases plasma arginine concentration in adults," Nutrition. 2007 Mar.; 23(3): 261-266.

Cook, N., et al. "Joint effects of sodium and potassium intake on subsequent cardiovascular disease: the trials of hypertension prevention follow-up study," Archives of Internal Medicine. 2009 Jan.; 169(1): 32-40.

Costa, A.P., et al. "High sodium intake adversely affects oxidative-inflammatory response, cardiac remodelling and mortality after myocardial Infarction," Atherosclerosis. 2012 May; 222(1): 284-291.

Crowell, P. and M. Gould. "Chemoprevention and therapy of cancer by d-limonene," Critical Reviews in Oncogenesis. 1994; 5(1): 1-22.

Danby, F.W. "Nutrition and aging skin: sugar and glycation," Clinics in Dermatology. 2010 Jul.-Aug.; 28(4): 409-411.

De Sprit S., et al. "An encapsulated fruit and vegetable juice concentrate increases skin microcirculation in healthy women," Skin Pharmacology and Physiology. 2012; 25: 2-8.

Delarue, J., et al. "Fish oil prevents the adrenal activation elicited by mental stress in healthy men," Diabetes & Metabolism. 2003 Jun.; 29(3): 289-295.

"Diet starts today…and ends on Friday: how we quickly slip back into bad eating habits within a few days," Daily Mail, September 16, 2013.

Dimitrios, B. "Sources of natural phenolic antioxidants," Trends in Food Science & Technology. 2006 Sep.; 17(9): 505-512.

Ditre, C. "Glycolic acid peels," Dermatologic Therapy. 2000 Apr.; 13(2): 165-172.

Ditre, C. "Glycolic acid peels," Dermatologic Therapy. 2000 Apr.; 13(2): 165-172.

Dmitrieva, N. and M. Burg. "Elevated sodium and dehydration stimulate inflammatory signaling in endothelial cells and promote atherosclerosis," PLoS ONE. 2015 Jun.; 10(6): e0128870.

Drewnowski, A., et al. "Reducing the sodium-potassium ratio in the US diet: a challenge for public health," The American Journal of Clinical Nutrition. 2012 Aug.; 96(2): 439-444.

Drummond, E.M., et al., "Inhibition of proinflammatory biomarkers in THP1 macrophages by polyphenols derived from chamomile, meadowsweet and willow bark," Phytotherapy Research. 2013 Apr.; 27(4): 588-594.

Durai, P.C., et al. "Aging in elderly: chronological versus photoaging," Indian Journal of Dermatology. 2012 Sep.-Oct.; 57(5): 343–352.

English, J. and H. Cass. "The collagen connection," Nutrition Review. 2013 Apr.

Epstein, J., et al. "Curcumin as therapeutic agent: the evidence from in vitro, animal and human studies," British Journal of Nutrition. 2010 Jun.; 103(11): 1545-1557.

Fasset, R. and J. Coombes. "Astaxanthin, oxidative stress, inflammation and cardiovascular disease," Future Cardiology. 2009; 4(3): 333-342.

Fisher, G.J. "The pathophysiology of photoaging of the skin," Cutis. 2005 Feb.; 75(2 Supp.): 5-8.

Flore, R., et al. "Something more to say about calcium homeostasis: the role of vitamin K2 in vascular calcification and osteoporosis," European Review for Medical and Phramacological Sciences. 2013 Sep.; 17(18): 2433-2440.

Fore-Pfliger, J. "The epidermal skin barrier: implication for the wound care practitioner, part I," Wound Care Journal. 2004 Oct.; 417-425.

Geronikaki, A. and A. Gavalas. "Antioxidants and inflammatory disease: synthetic and natural antioxidants with anti-inflammatory activity," Combinatorial Chemistry & High Throughput Screening. 2006 Jul.; 9(6): 425-442.

Gerster, H. "Can adults adequately convert alpha-linolenic acid (18:3n-3) to eicosapentaenoic acid (20:5n-3) and docosahexaenoic acid (22:6n-3)?" International Journal Vitamin Nutrition Research. 1998; 68(3): 159-73.

Ghanbari, R., et al. "Valuable nutrients and functional bioactives in different parts of olive (olea europea l.) – a review," International Journal of Molecular Sciences. 2012; 13(3): 3291-3340.

Gonzalez-Gomez, D., et al. "Detection and quantification of melatonin and serotonin in eight sweet cherry cultivars (prunus avium L.)," European Food Research and Technology. 2009 Jun.; 229(2): 223-229.

Graf, E. "Antioxidant potential of ferulic acid," Free Radical Biology and Medicine. 1992 Oct.; 13(4): 435-448.

Green, R., et al. "Common tea formulations modulate in vitro digestive recovery of green tea catechins," Molecular Nutrition and Food Research. 2007 Sep.; 51(9): 1152-1162.

Grosso, G., et al. "Red orange: experimental models and epidemiological evidence of its benefits on human health," Oxidative Medicine and Cellular Longevity. 2013: 1-11.

Gu, Y., et al. "Dietary inflammation factor rating system and risk of Alzheimer's disease in elders," Alzheimer Disease & Associated Disorders. 2011 Apr.-Jun.; 25(2): 149-154.

Guimaraes, R., et al. "Targeting excessive free radicals with peels and juices of citrus fruits: grapefruit, lemon, lime and orange," Food and Chemical Toxicology. 2010 Jan.; 48(1): 99-106.

Haleblian, G.E., et al. "Assessment of citrate concentrates in citrus fruit-based juices and beverages: implications for management of hypocitraturic nephrolithiasis," Journal of Endourology. 2008 Jun.; 22(6): 1359-1366.

Hallberg, L., et al. "The role of vitamin C in iron absorption," International Journal of Vitamin and Nutrition Research. 1989; 30: 103-108.

Halprin, K. "Epidermal 'turnover time' – a re-examination," British Journal of Dermatology. 1972 Jan.; 86(1): 14-19.

Hamalainen, L., et al. "Synthesis and degradation of type I procollagen mRNAs in cultured human skin fibroblasts and the effect of cortisol," The Journal of Biological Chemistry. 1985 Jan.; 260: 720-725.

Hamm, T. 365 Ways to Live Cheap. Adams Media, 2008.

Harris, M. and R. Shipstova. "Consumer demand for convenience foods: demographics and expenditures," Journal of Food Distribution and Research. 2007 Nov.; 38(3): 22-36.

He, F., et al. "Beneficial effects of potassium on human health," Physiologia Plantarum. 2008 Aug.; 133(4): 725-735.

Heffernan, T., et al. "ATR-Chk1 pathway inhibition promotes apoptosis after UV treatment in primary human keratinocytes: potential basis for the UV protective effects of caffeine," Journal of Investigative Dermatology. 2009; 129: 1805-1815.

Heinrich, U., et al. "Green tea polyphenols provide photoprotection, increase microcirculation, and modulate skin properties of women," The Journal of Nutrition, 2011 Jun.; 141(6): 1202-1208.

Hipkiss, A.R. "Carnosine, a protective ,anti-ageing peptide?" Cell Biology. 1998 Aug.; 30(8): 863-868.

Hou, J.P., et al. "Isolation of some compounds from nutmeg and their antioxidant activities," Czech Journal of Food Science. 2012; 30(2): 164-170.

Howatson, G., et al. "Effects of tart cherry juice (prunus cerasus) on melatonin levels and enhanced sleep quality," European Journal of Nutrition. 2012 Dec.; 51(8): 909-916.

Hseu, Y., et al. "Ellagic acid protects human keratinocyte (HaCaT) cells against UVA-induced oxidative stress and apoptosis through the upregulation of the HO-1 and Nrf-2 antioxidant genes," Food and Chemical Toxicology. 2012 May; 50(5): 1245-1255.

Hsieh, T.H., et al. "Phthalates induce proliferation and invasiveness of estrogen receptor-negative breast cancer through the AhR/HDAC6/c-Myc signaling pathway," The Journal of the Federation of American Societies for Experimental Biology. 2012 Feb.; 26(2): 778-787.

Huber, M., et al. "Organic food and impact on human health: assessing the status quo and prospects of research," NJAS-Wageningen Journal of Life Sciences. 2011 Dec.; 58(3-4): 103-109.

Jacob, R., et al. "Consumption of cherries lowers plasma urate in healthy women," The Journal of Nutrition. 2003 Jun.; 133(6): 1826-1829.

James, William D., et al. Andrews' Diseases of the Skin: Clinical Dermatology, 12th Edition. Elsevier; 2016.

Jeon, J., et al. "Simultaneous determination of arbutin and its decomposed product hydroquinone in whitening creams using high-performance liquid chromatography with photodiode array detection: effect of temperature and pH on decomposition," International Journal of Cosmetic Science. 2015.

Jolly, H., et al. "Impact of warm compresses on local injection-site reactions with self-administered glatiramer acetate," Journal of Neuroscience Nursing. 2008 Aug.; 40(4): 232-240.

Joubert, E. and D. Ferreira. "Antioxidants of rooibos tea – a possible explanation for its health promoting properties?" The SA Journal of Food Science and Nutrition. 1996; 8(3): 79-83.

Jugdaohsing, R. "Silicon and bone health," Journal of Nutrition, Health & Aging. 2007 Mar.; 11(2): 99-110.

Kapoor, S. and S. Saraf. "Assessment of viscoelasticity and hydration effect of herbal moisturizers using bioengineering techniques," Pharmacognosy Magazine. 2010 Oct.-Dec.; 6(24): 298-304.

Kaur, J., et al. "Herbal medicines: possible risks and benefits," American Journal of Phytomedicine. 2013; 1(2): 226-239.

Kelley, D., et al. "Consumption of bing sweet cherries lowers circulating concentrations of inflammation markers in healthy men and women," The Journal of Nutrition. 2006 Apr.; 136(4): 981-986.

Khatum, M., et al. "Effect of thermal treatment on radical-scavenging activity of some spices," Food Science and Technology Research. 2006; 12(3): 178-185.

Kim, C. "Capsaicin exhibits anti-inflammatory property by inhibiting IkB-a degradation in LPS-stimulated peritoneal macrophages," Cell Signal. 2003 Mar.; 15(3): 299-306.

Kim, J.E., et al. "Effects of egg consumption on carotenoid absorption from co-consumed, raw vegetables," The American Journal of Clinical Nutrition. 2015; ajcn111062.

King, D., et al. "Trends I dietary fiber intake in the United States, 1999-2008," Journal of the Academy of Nutrition and Dietetics. 2012 May; 112(5): 642-648.

Kochhar, K.P. "Dietary spices in health and diseases: I," Indian Journal of Physiology and Pharmacology. 2008 Apr.-Jun.; 52(2): 106-122.

Koo, M. and C. Cho. "Pharmacological effects of green tea on the gastrointestinal system," European Journal of Pharmacology. 2004 Oct.; 500(1-3): 177-185.

Kris-Etherton, P., et al. "Fish consumption, fish oil, omega-3 fatty acids, and cardiovascular disease," Circulation. 2002; 106: 2747-2757.

Lantz, R., et al. "The effect of turmeric extracts on inflammatory mediator production," Phytomedicine. 2005 Jun.; 12(6-7): 445-452.

Latreille, J., et al. "Dietary monounsaturated fatty acids intake and risk of skin photoaging," PLoS ONE. 2012 Sep.; 7(9): e44490.

Lee, A., et al. "Consumption of tomato products with olive oil but not sunflower oil increases the antioxidant activity of plasma," Free Radical Biology and Medicine. 2000 Nov.; 29(10): 1051-1055.

Lephart, E. "Human skin gene expression, attributes of botanicals: angelica sinensis, a soy extract, equol and its isomers and resveratrol," Gene Technology. 2015 Apr.; 4(2): 119-127.

Lieberman, S. The Gluten Connection: How Gluten Sensitivity May Be Sabotaging Your Health and What You Can Do to Take Control Now. Rodale Books. 2006.

Lin, F., et al. "Ferulic acid stabilizes a solution of vitamins C and E and doubles its photoprotection of skin," Journal of Investigative Dermatology. 2005; 125: 826-832.

Liu, R. "Health benefits of fruit and vegetables are from additive and synergistic combinations of phytochemicals," The American Journal of Clinical Nutrition. 2003 Sep.; 78(3): 517S-520S.

Liu, R. "Potential synergy of phytochemicals in cancer prevention: mechanism of action," The Journal of Nutrition. 2004 Dec.; 134(12): 3479S-3485S.

Lodish, H., et al. Molecular Cell Biology, 4th Edition. W.H. Freeman; 2000.

Lonnerdal, B. "Dietary factors influencing zinc absorption," The Journal of Nutrition. 2000 May; 130(5): 1378S-1383S.

Luqman, S. et al. "Protection of lipid peroxidation and carbonyl formation in proteins by capsaicin in human erythrocytes subjected to oxidative stress," Phytotherapy Research. 2006 Apr.; 20(4): 303-306.

Magner, J., et al., "Human exposure to pesticides from food," Swedish Environmental Research Institute: Report No. U 5080. 2015.

Martinez-Cruz, O., et al. "Phytochemical profile and nutraceutical potential of chia seeds (salvia hispanica l.) by liquid chromatography," Journal of Chromatography A. 2014 Jun.; 1346: 43-48.

Masibo, M., et al. "Major mango polyphenols and their potential significance to human health," Comprehensive Reviews in Food Science and Food Safety. 2008 Oct.; 7(4): 309-319.

McClain, G., et al. "The role of polyphenols in skin health," Bioactive Dietary Factors and Plant Extracts in Dermatology Nutrition and Health. 2013: 169-175.

McKay, D. and J. Blumberg. "A review of the bioactivity and potential health benefits of peppermint tea (mentha piperita l.)," Phytotherapy Research. 2006 Aug.; 20(8): 619-633.

Meschino, J.P. "Essential fatty acid supplementation improves skin texture and overall health," Dynamic Chiropractic. 2003 Sep.

Mikirova, N., et al. "Circulating endothelial progenitor cells: a new approach to anti-aging medicine?" Journal of Translational Medicine. 2009 Dec.; 7: 106-117.

Milde, J., et al. "Synergistic effects of phenolics and carotenoids on human low-density lipoprotein oxidation," Molecular Nutrition and Food Research. 2007 Aug.; 51(8): 956-961.

Mozaffarian, R., et al. "Identifying whole grain foods: a comparison of different approaches for selecting more healthful whole grain products," Public Health Nutrition. 2013 Dec.; 16(12): 2255-2264.

Murakami, H., et al. "Importance of amino acid composition to improve skin collagen protein synthesis rates in UV-irradiated mice," Amino Acids. 2012 Jun.; 42(6): 2481-2489.

Ndiaye, M., et al. "The grape antioxidant resveratrol for skin disorders: promise, prospects, and challenges," Archives of Biochemistry and Biophysics. 2011 Apr.; 508(2): 164-170.

Nichols, P., et al. "Readily available sources of long-chain omega-3 oils: is farmed Australian seafood a better source of the good oil than wild-caught seafood?" Nutrients. 2014; 6(3): 1063-1079.

Niki, E., et al. "Ineraction among vitamin C, vitamin E, and beta-carotene." American Journal of Clinical Nutrition. 1995 Dec.; 62(6 Supp.): 1322S-1326S.

Noor, N.M, et al. "The effect of virgin coconut oil loaded solid lipid particles (VCO-SLPs) on skin hydration and skin elasticity," Journal Teknologi. 2013 May; 62(1): 39-43.

Marina, A.M., et al. "Antioxidant capacity and phenolic acids of virgin coconut oil," International Journal of Food Sciences and Nutrition. 2009; 60(Supp. 2): 114-123.

Nsimba, R.Y., et al. "Ecdysteroids act as inhibitors of calf skin collagenase and oxidative stress," Journal of Biochemical and Molecular Toxicology. 2008 Jul./Aug.; 22(4): 240-250.

Nuutila, A.M., et al. "Comparison of antioxidant activities of onion and garlic extracts by inhibition of lipid peroxidation and radical scavenging activity," Food Chemistry. 2003 Jun.; 81(4): 485-493.

Ohla, S., et al. "Chip electrophoresis of active banana ingredients with label-free detection utilizing deep UV native fluorescence and mass spectrometry," Analytical and Bioanalytical Chemistry. 2011 Feb.; 339(5): 1853-1857.

Oliveira, M.C., et al. "Acute and sustained inflammation and metabolic dysfunction induced by high refined carbohydrate-containing diet in mice," Obesity. 2013 Sep.; 21(9): E396-E406.

Pallela, R. "Antioxidants from marine organisms and skin care," Systems Biology of Free Radicals and Antioxidants. 2014 May; 166: 3771-3783.

Pan, S., et al. "Parabens and human epidermal growth factor receptor ligands cross-talk in breast cancer cells," Environmental Health Perspectives. 2015.

Panchatcharam, M., et al. "Curcumin improves wound healing by modulating collagen and decreasing reactive oxygen species," Molecular and Cellular Biochemistry. 2006 Mar.; 290(1): 87-96.

Pandel, R., et al. "Skin photoaging and the role of antioxidants in its prevention," ISRN Dermatology, 2013.

Pandjaitan, N., et al. "Antioxidant capacity and phenolic content of spinach as affected by genetics and maturation," Journal of Agricultural and Food Chemistry. 2005 Nov.; 53(22): 8618-8623.

Parengkuan, L., et al. "Anti-glycation activity of various fruits," Anti-Aging Medicine. 2013; 10(4): 70-76.

Patil, M., et al. "Pharmacological evaluation of ameliorative effect of aqueous extract of cucumis sativus l. fruit formulation on wound healing in wistar rats," Chronicles of Young Scientists. 2011; 2(4): 207-213.

Peres, P.S., et al. "Photoaging and chronological aging profile: understanding oxidation of the skin," Journal of Photochemistry and Photobiology B: Biology. 2011 May; 103(2): 93-97.

Perez-Sanchez, A., et al. "Protective effects of citrus and rosemary extracts on UV-induced damage in skin cell model and human volunteers," Journal of Photochemistry and Photobiology B: Biology. 2014 Jul.; 136: 12-18.

Poon, F, et al. "Mechanisms and treatments of photoaging," Photodermatology, Photoimmunology & Photomedicine. 2015 Mar.; 31(2): 65-74.

Poudyal, H. "Omega-3 fatty acids and metabolic syndrome: effects and emerging mechanisms of action," Progress in Lipid Research. 2011 Oct.; 50(4): 372-387.

Prakash, D. "Antioxidant and free radical scavenging activities of phenols from onion (allium cepa)," Food Chemistry. 2007; 102(4): 1389-1393.

Preuss, H.G., et al. "Whole cinnamon and aqueous extracts ameliorate sucrose-induced blood pressure elevations in spontaneously hypertensive rats," Journal of the American College of Nutrition. 2006; 25(2): 144-150.

Purba, M., et al. "Skin wrinkling: can food make a difference?" Journal of the American College of Nutrition. 2001; 20(1): 71-80.

Putnam, J., et al. "U.S. per capita food supply trends: more calories, refined carbohydrates, and fats," Food Review: The Magazine of Food Economics. 2002 Winter. 25(3): 2-15.

Rani, B., et al. "Invigorating efficacy of cucumis sativas for healthcare & radiance," International Journal of Chemistry and Pharmaceutical Sciences. 2014; 2(3): 737-744.

Razquin, C., et al. "A 3 years follow-up of a Mediterranean diet rich in virgin olive oil is associated with high plasma antioxidant capacity and reduced body weight gain," European Journal of Clinical Nutrition. 2009; 63: 1387-1393.

Reiter, R., et al. "Melatonin in walnuts: influence on levels of melatonin and total antioxidant capacity of blood," Nutrition. 2005 Sep.; 21(9): 920-924.

Riedeger, N., et al. "A systemic review of the roles of n-3 fatty acids in health and disease," Journal of the American Dietetic Association. 2009 Apr.; 109(4): 668-679.

Rittie, L., et al. "Natural and sun-induced aging of human skin," Cold Spring Harbor Perspectives in Medicine. 2015 Jan.; 5(9): a015370.

Rizwan, M., et al. "Tomato paste rich in lycopene protects against cutaneous photodamage in humans in vivo: a randomized controlled trial" British Journal of Dermatology. 2011 Jan; 164(1): 154-162.

Roh, E., et al. "Molecular mechanisms of green tea polyphenols with protective effects against skin photoaging," Critical Reviews in Food Science and Nutrition. 2015.

Rolstad, B., et al. "Relating knowledge of anatomy and physiology of the skin to peristomal skin care," World Council of Enterostomal Therapists Journal. 2012 Jan.-Mar.; 32: 4-10.

Ros, E., et al. "Fatty acid composition of nuts – implications for cardiovascular health," British Journal of Nutrition. 2006 Nov.; 96 (Supp. 2): S29-S35.

Rosenblat, G., et al. "Polyhydroxylated fatty alcohols derived from avocado suppress inflammatory response and provide non-sunscreen protection against UV-induced damage in skin cells," Archives of Dermatological Research. 2011 May; 303(4): 239-246.

Saija, A., et al. "In vitro and in vivo evaluation of caffeic and ferulic acids as topical photoprotective agents," International Journal of Pharmaceutics. 2000 Apr.; 199(1): 39-47.

Sampath Kumar, K.P., et al. "Traditional and medicinal uses of banana," Journal of

Pharmacognosy and Phytochemistry. 2012; 1(3): 51-63.

Sampson, H. and C. Marshall. "Food hypersensitivity and atopic dermatitis: evaluation of 113 patients," The Journal of Pediatrics. 1985 Nov.; 107(5): 669-675.

Schloms, L., et al. "Rooibos influences glucocorticoid levels and steroid ratios in vivo and in vitro: a natural approach in the management of stress and metabolic disorders?" Molecular Nutrition & Food Research. 2014 Mar.; 58(3): 537-549.

Schloms, L., et al. "The influence of aspalathus linearis (rooibos) and dihydrochalcones on adrenal steroidogenesis: quantification of steroid intermediates and end products in H295R cells," The Journal of Steroid Biochemistry and Molecular Biology. 2012 Feb.; 128(3-5): 128-138.

Seeram, N., et al. Antioxidant Measurement and Applications. ACS Symposium Series, Vol. 956, 2009: Chapter 21: "Impact of berry phytochemicals on human health: effects beyond antioxidation," pp. 326-336.

Seo, D., et al. "Biotechnological production of arbutins (a- and B-arbutins), skin lightening agents, and their derivatives," Applied Microbiology and Biotechnology. 2012 Sep.; 95(6): 1417-1425.

Shan, B., et al. "Antioxidant capacity of 26 spice extracts and characterization of their phenolic constituents," Journal of Agricultural and Food Chemistry. 2005 Sep.; 53(20): 7749-7759.

Sheridan, M., et al. "Pistachio nut consumption and serum lipid levels," Journal of the American College of Nutrition. 2007; 26(2): 141-148.

Shoba, G., et al. "Influence of piperine on the pharmacokinetics of curcumin in animals and human volunteers," Planta Medica. 1998 May; 64(4): 353-356.

Shokri Mashhadi, N., et al. "Anti-oxidative and anti-inflammatory effects of ginger in health and physical activity: review of current evidence," International Journal of Preventive Medicine. 2013 Apr.; 4(Supp. 1): S36-S42.

Shonagh, W. "Body matters: skin hygiene: think you know all about skin…think again," PS Post Script. 2015 Feb.; 30-31.

Shukla, Y., et al. "Cancer preventive properties of ginger: a brief review," Food and Chemical Toxicology. 2007 May; 45(5): 683-690.

Sikora, E., et al. "Composition and antioxidant activity of kale (brassica oleracea l. var. acephala) raw and cooked," ACTA Scientarium Polonorum Technologia Alimentaria. 2012; 11(3): 239-248.

Silalahi, J. "Anticancer and health protective properties of citrus fruit components," Asia Pacific Journal of Clinical Nutrition. 2002 Mar.; 11(1): 79-84.

Simopoulos, A.P. "The importance of the ratio of omega-6/omega-3 essential fatty acids," Biomedicine Pharmacotherapy. 2002 Oct.; 56(8): 365-379.

Simpson, R., et al. "Exercise and the aging immune system," Aging Research Reviews. 2012 Jul.; 11(3): 404-420.

Smirnoff, N. "Plant resistance to environmental stress," Current Opinion in Biotechnology. 1998 Apr.; 9(2): 214-219.

Solomon, A. "Antioxidant activities and anthocyanin content of fresh fruits of common fig (ficus carica l.)," Journal of Agricultural and Food Chemistry. 2006; 54(20): 7717-7723.

Song, W., et al. "Cellular antioxidant activity of common vegetables," Journal of Agricultural and Food Chemistry. 2010; 58(11): 6621-6629.

Sosa, M., et al. "Evaluation of the topical anti-inflammatory activity of ginger dry extracts from solutions and plasters," Planta Medica. 2007; 73(15): 1525-1530.

Sripanyakorn, S., et al. "The comparative absorption of silicon from different foods and food supplements," British Journal of Nutrition. 2009 Sep.; 102(6): 825-834.

Stahl, W., et al. "Carotenoids and flavonoids contribute to nutritional protection against skin damage from sunlight," Molecular Biology. 2007 Sep.; 37(1): 26-30.

Steptoe, A., et al. "The effect of tea on psychophysiological stress responsivity and post-stress recovery: a randomised double-blind trial," Psychopharmacology. 2007 Jan.: 190(1): 81-89.

Stevenson, D., et al. "Oil and tocopherol content and composition of pumpkin seed oil in 12 cultivars," Journal of Agricultural and Food Chemistry. 2007; 55(10): 4005-4013.

Su, L., et al. "Total phenolic contents, chelating capacities, and radical-scavenging properties of black peppercorn, nutmeg, rosehip, cinnamon and oregano leaf," Food Chemistry. 2007; 100(3): 990-997.

Suhaj, M. "Spice antioxidants isolation and their antiradical activity: a review," Journal of Food Composition and Analysis. 2006 Sep.-Nov.; 19(6-7): 531-537.

Suo, M., et al. "Phenolic lipid ingredients from cashew nuts," Journal of Natural Medicines. 2012 Jan.; 66(1): 133-139.

Tabas, I. and C. Glass, "Anti-inflammatory therapy in chronic disease: challenges and opportunities," Science. 2013 Jan.; 339(6116): 166-172.

Talbott, S. Cortisol Control and the Beauty Connection. Ch. 4: "Inside-out help for wrinkles, acne, and 'problem' skin," Hunter House Publishers, Inc., 2007.

Tanase, C., et al. "Sodium and potassium in composite food samples from the Canadian total diet study," Journal of Food Composition and Analysis. 2011 Mar.; 24(2): 237-243.

Thompson, A. "Acne," The Journal of the American Medical Association. 2015 Feb.; 313(6): 640.

Tomaino, A., et al. "Antioxidant activity and phenolic profile of pistachio (pistacia vera l., variety bronte) seeds and skins," Biochimie. 2010 Sep.; 92(9): 1115-1122.

USDA Nutrition and Your Health: Dietary Guidelines for Americans, Appendix G-2: Original Food Guide Pyramid Patterns and Description of USDA Analyses, Addendum A: EPA and DHA Content of Fish Species.

Vasanthi, H.R., et al. "Potential health benefits of broccoli – a chemico-biological overview," Mini-Reviews in Medicinal Chemistry. 2009 Jun.; 9(6): 749-759.

Vega-Galvez, A., et al. "Nutrition facts and functional potential of quinoa (chenopodium quinoa willd.), an ancient Andean grain: a review," Journal of the Science of Food Agriculture. 2010 Dec.; 90(15): 2541-2547.

Veloso, C., et al. "Hydroethanolic extract of pyrostegia venusta (ker gawl.) miers flowers improves inflammatory and metabolic dysfunction induced by high-refined carbohydrate diet," Journal of Ethnopharmacology. 2014 Jan.; 151(1): 722-728.

Walburn, J., et al. "Psychological stress and wound healing in humans: a systematic review and meta-analysis," Journal of Psychosomatic Research. 2009 Sep.; 67(3): 253-271.

Wall, R., et al. "Fatty acids from fish: the anti-inflammatory potential of long-chain omega-3 fatty acids," Nutrition Reviews. 2010; 68(5): 280-289.

Wang, S., et al. "Synergistic, additive, and antagonistic effects of food mixtures on total antioxidant capacities," Journal of Agricultural and Food Chemistry. Ya 2011 Jan.; 59(3): 960-968.

Watts, D. "The nutritional relationships of manganese," Journal of Orthomolecular Medicine. 1990; 5(4): 219-222.

Weinstein, G., et al. "Cell proliferation in normal epidermis," Journal of Investigative Dermatology. 1984; 82: 623-628.

Whitehead, R., et al. "You are what you eat: within-subject increases in fruit and vegetable consumption confer beneficial skin-color changes," PLoS ONE. 2012; 7(3): e32988.

Wilson, E., et al. "Antioxidant, anti-inflammatory, and antimicrobial properties of garlic and onions," Nutrition & Food Science. 2007; 37(3): 178-183.

Wolf, R., et al. (Eds.). Emergency Dermatology. Cambridge University Press. 2011: 321-322.

Worthington, V. "Nutritional quality of organic versus conventional fruits, vegetables, and grains," The Journal of Alternative and Complementary Medicine. 2001 Apr.; 7(2): 161:173.

Yamamoto, Y., et al. "Effects of alpha-hydroxy acids on the human skin of Japanese subjects: the rationale for chemical peeling," Journal of Dermatology. 2006 Jan.; 33(1): 16-22.

Yanishlieva, N., et al. "Natural antioxidants from herbs and spices," European Journal of Lipid Science and Technology. 2006 Sep.; 108(9): 776-793.

Zhang, J. and J. An. "Cytokines, inflammation and pain," International Anesthesiology Clinics. 2007 Spring; 45(2): 27-37.

ABOUT THE AUTHOR

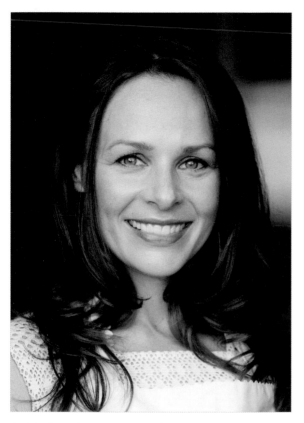

Michelle Lee is author of *Living Luxe Gluten Free*, which was nominated for the James Beard Book Award for Focus on Health. Her book has been praised as "exceptional...beautiful...impressive" (*Gluten Free & More Magazine*), "adventurous... useful" (*Publishers Weekly*), "upscale...luxurious" (*Simply Gluten Free Magazine*) and "highly recommended" (*Midwest Book Review*).

Ms. Lee is featured on KLRR's morning show where she shares healthy living tips and recipes on "Delicious Dishes with Michelle Lee."

In addition to her culinary work, Ms. Lee is an award-winning economics and business consultant who has been featured in various publications, including *Forbes*, for her research. Ms. Lee holds a degree in economics and an MBA.

Aside from her passions for healthy living and economics, Ms. Lee is a fitness enthusiast, who has placed in distance running competitions on two continents and has received recognitions including top finisher medals in 10k races, qualification for the Boston Marathon, the Archie Griffin Sportsmanship Award, and MVP of varsity cheerleading. In 1998, she was crowned Miss Teen Columbus.

Michelle presently resides in Oregon with her family and rescued German Shepherd-Border Collie dog.

NOTES

NOTES

NOTES